The HEADACHE HEALER'S HANDBOOK

A Holistic, Hands-On Somatic Self-Care Program for Headache and Migraine Relief and Prevention

Jan Mundo, CMSC, CMT

Illustrations by Jan Mundo

Foreword by Alexander Mauskop, MD

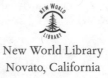

New World Library
Novato, California

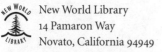

New World Library
14 Pamaron Way
Novato, California 94949

Illustrations by Jan Mundo
Text design by Tona Pearce Myers

Library of Congress Cataloging-in-Publication Data
Names: Mundo, Jan, [date] author.
Title: The headache healer's handbook : a holistic, hands-on somatic self-care program
    for headache and migraine relief and prevention / Jan Mundo, CMSC, CMT.
Description: Novato, California : New World Library, [2018] | Includes bibliographical
    references and index.
Identifiers: LCCN 2017054983 (print) | LCCN 2018001334 (ebook) | ISBN 9781608685141
    (Ebook) | ISBN 9781608685134 (alk. paper)
Subjects: LCSH: Headache—Alternative treatment. | Holistic medicine. |
    Headache—Prevention.
Classification: LCC RB128 (ebook) | LCC RB128 .M86 2018 (print) | DDC
    616.8/491—dc23
LC record available at https://lccn.loc.gov/2017054983

First printing, May 2018
ISBN 978-1-60868-513-4
Ebook ISBN 978-1-60868-514-1
Printed in Canada on 100% postconsumer-waste recycled paper

New World Library is proud to be a Gold Certified Environmentally Responsible Publisher. Publisher certification awarded by Green Press Initiative.
www.greenpressinitiative.org

10   9   8   7   6   5   4   3   2   1

*To my inspirational teachers in the arts, healing,
and life, who saw me and kindly lit the way.
Your impact is everlasting.*

Contents

Part Three. Creating Balance through Awareness

Part Four. Hands On: The Healing Power of Touch

Part Five. The Deeper Realms of Headache

Foreword

Headaches afflict close to half of the U.S. population, with 40 million suffering from migraines, which can be very disabling. Many books have been written for the general public, including two of my own, but Jan Mundo's *Headache Healer's Handbook* brings a unique perspective to this problem.

When I treat patients in the office, they are usually reassured by the fact that I am also a migraine sufferer, and so it is with Jan's book — she knows firsthand what it feels like to have a migraine. More importantly, she has discovered ways to relieve her own attacks and those of countless other migraineurs.

Like Jan, I am a big proponent of nondrug treatments, and this is what she details in her book. I also like her hands-on approach, both literally and figuratively. Psychologists have proven that active treatments, where people are doing things to improve their condition, are much more effective than passive treatments, such as massage, chiropractic, and acupuncture, where things are done to them. This leads to the transfer from an external locus of control to an internal locus of control or, in other words, a shift from being a passive and helpless victim of external circumstances to being an active participant in the events with a significant degree of control.

Jan begins with the basics — identifying your type of headache and finding possible triggers that make your headaches worse. She recommends at least one visit to the doctor to confirm the diagnosis. This is important not because a brain tumor or an aneurysm is likely to be found (since those are very rare), but because a routine blood test could detect a magnesium or thyroid deficiency, anemia, or another medical problem that could be contributing to headaches.

Once your diagnosis is confirmed, with Jan's help you can take an inventory of your diet, sleeping habits, physical environment, and posture to try to find triggers, which can be corrected. Then Jan recommends breathing exercises, which to me have echoes of the Feldenkrais Method; becoming aware of how you breathe can improve not only your breathing itself but also the movements of your chest, your spine, and the rest of your body.

In chapter 12, "Being Still: Mindfulness and Headaches," Jan describes another powerful tool in combating headaches as well as many other physical and mental ailments. Yes, everyone is talking about the proven benefits of meditation, but it is surprising how few people actually practice it.

Chapter 13, "Posture, Ergonomics, and Sleep," is followed by a chapter on physical exercise, which is proven not only to be good for you but to specifically reduce the frequency and the severity of headaches.

A large portion of the book is devoted to the Mundo Method, Jan's unique hands-on therapy, which she developed to treat her own headaches and which has helped many other sufferers she has worked with. The healing power of touch is scientifically proven to dramatically improve outcomes in premature babies, and without a doubt, it can also be harnessed to relieve a variety of headache conditions. Just follow Jan's advice, and watch your headaches go away.

— Alexander Mauskop, MD
Director, New York Headache Center
Professor of Clinical Neurology, SUNY, Downstate Medical Center

Preface

I became a healer by accident — at least, I didn't plan it.

In 1970, I intuitively began developing a hands-on method of headache and migraine relief. By placing my hands on someone's head, including my own, I could feel the headache (or *palpate* it, in medical terminology), work with its sensations, and stop it cold.

My clients swear I have magical hands, because I can relieve their headaches and migraines on the spot and halt the horrible symptoms that accompany their pain. I've relieved thousands of headaches with my protocol, but my work goes beyond that: I teach people how to heal *themselves*. I didn't envision this path, but the process was so compelling that it became my passion and life's work.

My Headache Story

My mom had severe migraines. As a child, I would massage away the knots and "spurs" from her shoulders and upper back. "Right there. Oh, that's good," she'd say. But mostly she would retreat to her darkened bedroom, cool washcloth on her forehead, and take a strong pain medication, which barely seemed to help. Until I developed migraines as an adult, I did not fully understand the severity of her pain.

My journey with headache healing began when I heard that you could relieve a headache by putting your hands on the front and back of the head. I gave it a try and, to my surprise, found I could stop a headache in its tracks. I started to experiment informally on people who had them, including myself, although during that time I didn't get them often because I was living a more natural lifestyle.

More accurately, I was living in a whole new world. Four years into my college education at the University of California, Berkeley, I had dropped out to join 250 other idealists following hippie guru Stephen Gaskin. Together we traveled, in a caravan of school buses, to the rolling fields of rural Tennessee, where we founded an intentional spiritual community, a commune really, called The Farm.

We were like modern-day pioneers. Dedicated to building a better world by "walking our talk," we bought 1,750 acres of land in the middle of nowhere and built a town, which grew to fifteen hundred residents. We raised, prepared, and preserved our food, eating a soy-based vegan diet with few sweets, no preservatives, and no alcohol. We had home births, assisted by midwives, and in the process we learned to trust the inherent wisdom of our bodies and the power of intention.

But even though we practiced meditation and followed Eastern as well as Western spiritual principles, collective living had its share of stressors. Thus, although my own headaches were rare back then, I got a lot of practice helping others with theirs.

In time, however, my situation changed. After leaving the community and returning to Los Angeles in 1985, I began getting frequent, debilitating migraines. Life was stressful. As a thirty-eight-year-old newly divorced mom of three kids who were experiencing big-city life for the first time, I was out on my own, struggling to support my family and starting a career in corporate America.

Several years later, I began waking up in the middle of the night, soaked in pools of perspiration, and I had hot flashes and mood swings during the day as well. I had no idea what was happening. Fortunately, my baby boomer generation often brought information into the public discourse that had previously been hidden and not discussed. This was especially true of issues involving women's bodies and hormonal life cycles. And then I learned that migraines often increase during perimenopause in women who are prone to them. Thus I was able to figure out that my strange symptoms indicated I was beginning perimenopause. I was astonished — I was only forty-two years old!

Seeking solutions to handle all of it — my stress, the perimenopause, and the migraines — I read a multitude of books by physicians, researchers, and wellness experts. These included mind-body books by physicians Herbert Benson, Deepak Chopra, Andrew Weil, and Jon Kabat-Zinn; women's health books by Christiane Northrup, MD, and Gail Sheehy; positive affirmation books by Shakti Gawain and Louise Hay; and headache books by Oliver Sacks, MD, and the physician-psychologist team of Roger K. Cady, MD, and Kathleen Farmer, PsyD. I attended lectures and monitored my body and habits.

Then I had a realization: in those months when I was eating regularly, drinking enough water, sleeping well, exercising, and remaining stress-aware, I did not get the blazing migraine that had become so predictable I could time my periods by it. I also noticed that my hot flashes were often preceded by angry or fearful thoughts. The connections between my mind, body, and health were becoming increasingly clear.

Life of a Headache Magnet

To my surprise, ever since I learned how to stop headaches on the spot in 1970, I seemed to become a magnet for people who had them. Wherever I went — work or job interview, party or family gathering, boutique or makeup counter — someone would inevitably complain to me, "Ugh, I've got such a headache! I have to [fill in the blank: take a break, go home, leave the party, lie down, take a pill...]."

So I would offer to help, saying, "I can stop your headache! All I'm going to do is put my hands on your head; just give me about five minutes." ("Really? Okay...") Lord knows why, but they trusted me. Slipping into the privacy of a nearby office, dressing room, the corner of a store or home, I would relieve the pain. Afterward, delighted and amazed, they would thank me and resume their activities, now pain-free. This occurred hundreds and hundreds of times without my understanding the process or knowing how pervasive the problem of headaches is.

Then in 1991, after twenty-one years of this informal experimentation, my path took an unexpected turn, and I made the decision to devote myself to a life in healing. I was working as a magazine advertising sales manager, finally at the top of my game and able to support my children, when I was suddenly laid off during our industry's annual trade show. I was devastated. But then just an hour later, in the middle of saying my goodbyes, I stopped a client's migraine — at her booth in the middle of the noisy Las Vegas Convention Center, packed with forty thousand people! I was surprised that my method worked even amid such chaos. A light bulb went off in my head, and I decided right then that I would teach others how to relieve their own pain.

The Scope of the Problem

In order to teach my healing method to others, I realized that not only would I need to become a keen observer of how it worked, but I would also need to learn all about headaches. I immersed myself in the literature, poring over consumer and medical books, peer-reviewed headache and neurology journals, countless articles, and research abstracts — until I began to understand the scope of the problem: there were millions of headache sufferers in the United States.

In 1992, there were an estimated 23.6 million migraineurs, of whom 11.3 million had moderate to severely debilitating migraines.[1] This population was "bedridden for about 3 million days per month and had an estimated 74.2 million days per year of restricted activity due to migraine," potentially costing businesses $1.4 billion in lost productivity annually.[2]

These staggering numbers are even higher today and, as in 1992, tell only half the story. Headache and migraine patients suffer for years, even decades, but not for lack of seeking a cure. Desperate for answers, most seek help over time from a variety of professionals, consulting with neurologists, pain specialists, psychiatrists, psychologists, dentists, orthodontists, optometrists, ENTs (ear, nose, and throat doctors), allergists, osteopaths, naturopaths, acupuncturists, chiropractors, homeopaths, nutritionists, yoga teachers, and mind-body practitioners, including biofeedback, physical, occupational, craniosacral, Reiki, and massage therapists.

And yet, after rounds of prescribed and over-the-counter medications and other therapies, millions of people still have millions of migraines. A particular drug might work at first but then lose its effectiveness. Patients who experience negative side effects from a medication or treatment discontinue it and switch to another therapy, thus beginning their search again. Prolonged reliance on one or a combination of medications results in increasingly frequent and intense episodes — and with their pain escalating, patients move on to another practitioner.

This miserable merry-go-round takes an emotional toll. Hope rises with the promise of each new, cutting-edge therapy, only to be dashed when it doesn't work. After years of suffering, headache patients become increasingly isolated, disillusioned, frustrated, and angry. They begin to accept the previously unimaginable prognosis that their migraines are incurable. Worn down and resigned to their fates, with hopes of a cure gone, many patients respond by giving up, doing nothing, falling into despair, or becoming drug-dependent, which still leaves them with cycles of chronic headaches and pain.

Headache Healing Confluences

These insights into the desperate world of headache sufferers made me more determined to teach my therapy. I thought: "There's all this suffering, and yet I can relieve a headache in minutes with my hands. I need to do what I can to bring my therapy out into the world."

But first, I had to determine whether anyone could do it, or if it was just *my* touch. I transcribed into words what I had been experiencing on the head and in my hands and created simple step-by-step instructions to describe the process. I asked several people with history of migraine to test my instructions, and my willing test subjects reported being able to "stop a headache in its tracks" or "back one down from escalating into a full-blown migraine." This was exciting!

In iterating the specifics of my method, I identified a fascinating cycle of sensations that occurred during the treatment. That is, all headaches had a predictable set of sensations that could be felt, altered, and released, and at each stage there were subtle, yet identifiable cues that, when complete, signaled relief. I used all these cues to codify my method into a protocol that included the focused concentration, or *mental push*, that seemed to shorten the treatment time.

Examining my method led me to a larger implication: not only did the headache resolve, but so did any associated migraine symptoms, such as nausea, disorientation, and sensitivity to light, sound, and odors. This signified an even bigger story: touch and concentration were producing neurological and physiological changes that were instantly affecting the brain, the pain, and the body's systems.

I met with medical, mind-body, and research professionals — brilliant and generous leaders in their respective fields — to introduce my work and find a path forward. In 1992, I graduated from Massage School of Santa Monica as a certified massage therapist, trained in myofascial and energy work, and opened my practice in California. My first patients were referred to me by UCLA associate clinical professor and neurologist Susan L. Perlman. Based on Dr. Perlman's follow-up comments — that her patients were able to successfully relieve but not prevent their headaches — I was inspired to design a program for prevention.

I attended medical research and scientific conferences and participated in early U.S. efforts to study complementary medicine. I went to the first National Institutes of Health (NIH) Office of Alternative Medicine Conference in Bethesda, Maryland, and to the NIH Clinical Research Training in San Francisco, California, in 1992. I attended four-day medical professional meetings, including "The Practicing Physician's Approach to the Difficult Headache Patient," sponsored by University of Chicago School of Medicine / Diamond Headache Clinic in 1992 and Annual Scientific Meetings of the American Headache Society in 1998, 1999, and 2001.

Attending my first medical conference was a fortunate coincidence. My dad, orthopedic surgeon Louis Spigelman, MD, had received an invitation to a headache conference and sent me instead. There, I was initially shocked to learn that most headache research was funded by the same pharmaceutical companies that develop and sell the drugs. They also sponsored significant portions of the conference — the doctors' breakfasts, coffee breaks, luncheons, dinners, galas, and educational seminars. I also got an unsettling glimpse into the competitive world of headache medicine when a neurologist who presented a lecture connecting food sensitivities and migraine was roundly criticized by his colleagues.

If medical professionals were so hard on each other and if money controlled the field, what chance did I stand? Escaping the lecture hall for the Palm Springs sunshine, I met the one person I needed to meet: neurologist and cluster headache specialist Dr. Lee Kudrow, Sr. I demonstrated my method to him, and he invited me to his office, where he encouraged me to continue my work and to further develop its mental focus component.

Personal health challenges again inadvertently shaped my healing path when I had a life-changing experience in a cathartic breathing workshop. During an unexpected emotional release in which I experienced a rush of memories, grief, and cognizance, my fifteen-year-long mysterious and disabling upper-back injury instantaneously began to dissipate. This was followed by months of feeling my fascia creak open like newly oiled rusty hinges. The entire experience left me with the tangible sense that our cells are holographic: they store our pain, emotions, thoughts, and memories — which are all bound together and can be released simultaneously.

I noticed similar experiences in my clients during the first year of my massage and headache practice. As they released tightness and pain, their emotions emerged. It was increasingly clear that their bodies held stories, which were related to their headaches. I was drawn to train in somatic (or "body-as-self") work to uncover and address the emotional roots of chronic pain and the unconscious, embodied patterns that hold it in place. Body-centered awareness helped my clients produce lasting change by connecting their headaches, habits, and underlying causes.

The Evolution of a Program

As a response to patients who still felt unheard or misunderstood after decades of chronic pain, stress, tension, fear, and frustration,

I designed a mind-body, self-care program that addressed the limitations of conventional medical treatment. Instead of taking medications for relief and prevention, clients would practice somatic awareness, breathing, meditation, aligned posture, self-massage, and hands-on headache therapy — along with headache-healthy diet, guidelines, and a diary for tracking everything. I hired expert consultants from the UCLA Statistical Biomathematical Consulting Clinic to refine my client questionnaires, and I began collecting intake and outtake data on my program.

I received certifications in Body-Centered and Conscious Relationship Transformation from the Hendricks Institute, Master Somatic Coaching and Bodywork from Strozzi Institute, and biofeedback training from Stens Corporation. I trained in Somatics and Trauma with Staci Haines / generationFIVE, studied developmental psychology at UC Berkeley Extension, and wove in courses in energy work, intuitive development, somatics, meditation, shamanism, writing, and expressive arts.

I began teaching my first medical center programs at Kaiser Permanente in 1995 after moving to the Bay Area. Fortuitously, my interviewer had divulged that she had been dealing with "a two-year migraine," so during the last five minutes of the interview, I stopped her pain. Thus, she subsequently facilitated my employment as a health educator at Kaiser Permanente, where I was also trained in course design.

I went on to teach my headache program to groups at medical centers, universities, corporations, community programs, and conferences, including Hill Physicians Medical Group, the UCSF Osher Center for Integrative Medicine, California Pacific Medical Center, the Institute for Health and Healing, UC Berkeley, Stanford University, Lockheed Martin, and Hewlett Packard. I gave workshops at the U.S. Association for Body-Psychotherapy Conference, the Association for Humanistic Psychology Conference, Integrative

Medicine Forums at UCSF Medical School and UC Berkeley, and the International Somatics Congress.

Then nurse practitioner candidates at Holy Names College in Oakland, California, contacted me and asked if I had data for a research study. (Oh, did I have data! Finally, I'd get to use the client self-report information I'd been collecting!) Thus in 2000, the Mundo Program was brought to light in a retrospective pilot study that looked at seventy-eight migraine patients who had completed the program through their HMOs. The study found that the patients were able to reduce their number of migraines by 41 percent and their use of relief medications by 52 percent upon completing a four-, five-, or six-week class (depending on the institution).

The results were remarkable, but especially because this was a brief training period — and the patients had a median of nineteen headache years (meaning some had them for less time and others had them for more), which is a lot. Also, notably, 97 percent of the participants reported feeling better about, more educated about, and in greater control of their migraines, whether or not they were still having them. The findings were published in *Cephalalgia*, the peer-reviewed international medical journal of headache, and presented in poster session at the 2001 International Headache Congress in New York City.[3]

This was exciting! At last I had independent verification that my program worked. Looking forward to sharing it with more people, I then created the first iteration of my book proposal, which has finally come to fruition as *The Headache Healer's Handbook*.

So welcome to my headache healer's world, where you put your hands on your head and use them like biofeedback sensors to stop your pain! Working with pain as sensations and solving headache mysteries is fascinating — and I'm delighted to share my healing secrets with you.

Introduction

The Headache Healer's Handbook presents the comprehensive Mundo Program for self-care relief and prevention in book form. In these pages, you will learn how to find the sources of your headache pain, prevent future attacks, and curb active headaches naturally — without having to resort to medications with their potential side effects.

Although comprehensive, this book is not one-size-fits-all. It coaches you step by step through an in-depth process of tracking down your triggers while addressing the unique challenges of conquering headaches and embracing self-care.

Tips and techniques alone cannot inspire people to make changes or sustain them. That's why this book embodies the *somatic experience*, a hallmark of the Mundo Program. Somatic self-care is a process of becoming aware of and working with the whole self — body, mind, emotions, and spirit. Gently and logically, the book will guide you inward to find and erase the underlying causes of your headaches, handle obstacles along the way, and move beyond a life defined by pain.

Parts of the Book and Program

Each section of the book addresses foundational skills and parts of the program that then prepare you for the next.

Part 1, "Entering In," provides the background to begin understanding the mind-body-headache connection and how to be successful with the plan. It introduces and defines the Mundo Program and starts your journey of looking at your headaches in a new light.

Part 2, "Handling Headache Triggers," turns you into a headache detective, out to track down your exact headache type and origins. It provides tools and skills to use throughout the program to identify and eliminate headache triggers in all areas of your life, with special attention devoted to migraine and diet.

Part 3, "Creating Balance through Awareness," guides you through a full stress-reduction program, including instruction and coaching in centered breathing, meditation, posture, and movement exercises. Its calming practices, everyday solutions, and gentle exercises help to create balance, prevent headaches, and promote overall health and well-being.

Part 4, "Hands On: The Healing Power of Touch," develops your kinesthetic abilities and shows in detail how to work directly with tension, holding, and pain in your shoulders, neck, head, and face — and to stop your headache or migraine on the spot.

Part 5, "The Deeper Realms of Headache," returns to somatics and how and why life experiences, including trauma, can be held in the body and perpetuate pain. Awareness exercises lead you inward to explore embodied responses, emotions in the body, and centering.

The conclusion, "Embodying Your New Life," is the completion segment of the program, where you identify, assess, and appreciate your progress. This final section calls you to envision beyond your headaches and pain and to create the vibrant, full, enjoyable life you have always wanted.

My client Michelle described her transformation this way:

After only a couple of months of learning and practicing the Mundo Program, things began to change. Not only did the headaches reduce in intensity and frequency, but my sleep patterns were better, stress levels were down, and physically I became much more comfortable in my body.

By the end of the program, I had learned how to stop a headache before it escalated, deal with it when I had one, and bounce back faster after it was over. The breathing, relaxation, and diet changes, along with applying Mundo Method therapy when necessary, have almost eliminated the migraines altogether.

I also have the added bonus of approaching my entire life in a different way. This change in my typical reaction to situations has been noted by relatives, friends, and coworkers. After over thirty years of struggle, I feel as if I have found a new lease on life.

It's Time!

Headache pain does not have to be the defining narrative of your life. You can create a different story, in which you are not the victim. You can overcome obstacles, learn lessons from them, and move on to fulfill your true life purpose.

As incredible as it might sound to you right now, you have the capacity to conquer your cycles of pain. It is possible to have a direct experience with your body that is pleasurable instead of painful. That is where we are headed together — and your intention, awareness, mind-body practices, healthy diet, powers of touch, and sensible choices will take you there.

Are you ready to take that journey from pain to vibrant health, guided by *The Headache Healer's Handbook*? Let's begin!

Part One

Entering In

1 Putting Relief in Your Hands

*D*o you remember your last severe migraine? If so, you would probably rather forget it if you could. If you've ever had one, then you know migraine's devastating, all-consuming misery. More than just pain, it puts you under its spell, possesses your entire being, and renders you a blob on the bed, unable to form a thought. All you can do is stay still and hope to quell the nausea and pounding — BA BOOM, BA BOOM, BA BOOM — that goes on and on, sometimes for days, even weeks.

Stumbling to the bathroom to find your rescue medication and hoping you don't throw up, you catch your face in the mirror and barely recognize yourself. As you make your way back to bed, you pray that the pill will stay down and take effect. Fear creeps in. Last time when the pain was this bad, you went to the emergency room for a shot of Demerol. You wonder if you should call your doctor now or suffer through it and wait until your next appointment?

What if there was another way — a completely different option? Imagine that you wake up with a splitting headache and give yourself a hands-on treatment that completely relieves your pain, nausea, vomiting, and other symptoms. In an hour or two, instead of days, your headache is gone, and your body recalibrates: your equilibrium returns, your face regains its color, and your eyes can tolerate the light. The jangling sounds and sickening odors that overwhelmed you just moments before have receded into the background.

Inhale. Exhale. Ah-h-h. You finally take a deep breath and let it go. You feel fine, your appetite returns, and you have a bite to eat. Soon everything is back to normal. You resume your day, and it's as if the migraine never happened. That night you sleep well, and you awake refreshed in the morning.

Can you imagine what it would be like to have that power over your headache or migraine pain? Or better yet: What if you could prevent your pain to begin with — and without medication or side effects? How would your life be different?

You're Not Alone

In the midst of a migraine, you might feel very alone — but you're not. Headaches are second only to back pain as the most common condition presented to doctors, and one in four U.S. households has a headache sufferer.[1]

Annually, an estimated 37 million people in the United States get migraines. Between one-half and two-thirds, or about 21 million, are women.[2] This disabling condition renders this population bedridden for 112 million days per year, which takes its toll on the business world too, costing companies $13 billion annually, $8 billion of which is attributed to missed workdays.[3] Adolescents and children are not immune either: Up to 10 percent of kids and teens, ages five to fifteen, and 28 percent of older teens, ages fifteen to nineteen, cope with migraine as one of their five most prevalent chronic conditions.[4]

Despite billions of healthcare dollars spent on medications and research, the exact causes of and solutions for migraine remain a mystery — and patients continue to suffer. Theories of pain, the brain, migraine causes, and who gets them and why have been studied, discussed, accepted, and rejected by clinicians, scientists, and researchers for the past century. They have examined blood flow, arterial and nerve inflammation, neurotransmitter activity, genetics, and more, but although science is certainly getting closer, no definitive mechanism has yet been found.

Doctors, books, and multiple online sources tell patients that migraines are forever and simply can't be cured, rendering famous the unnerving admonition: "You'll just have to learn to live with it." It seems unbelievable. Who wants to think they will always be in pain?

Not satisfied with sitting around, headache patients set out to find solutions. They seek help from neurologists, psychologists, and a variety of other specialists, who usually prescribe several medications to manage the pain and other symptoms — and even the primary medications' side effects. After much trial and error, they might seem to be doing better, but then the medications cease working, and so they begin their search for help again. Patients change therapies and doctors, add new specialists, and try complementary approaches, yet still they suffer.

Suzette, vice president of worldwide marketing for a high-tech company, had suffered from excruciating migraines since she was five years old. Through thirty years of dealing with pain, she had been "misdiagnosed, mismanaged, and misunderstood by traditional doctors, chiropractors, and alternative therapists." Hers was not the occasional headache that goes away with a couple of aspirin: she experienced the overwhelming combination of pain, nausea, and sensitivity to smells and light that is typical for migraine sufferers. Her search for relief was also typical:

> I had learned everything I could that science and medicine have uncovered about the diagnosis, treatment, and medications for migraine. My treatment over the years included almost every type of preventive medication and pain reliever,

from beta-blockers, epilepsy drugs, narcotic painkillers, and muscle relaxants to herbal remedies, supplements, and anti-nausea medication. I tried eliminating trigger foods, stressful situations, and schedule changes. In the last ten years, I was able to find one drug that worked well in stopping a headache if it was injected at the first sign of pain. Unfortunately, I knew my time was limited in using the drug because of its rebound qualities, and I wondered about possible effects on my heart as I grew older.

Suzette's story — of pain, frustration, and a remedy that complicates the original problem — is echoed by millions, and for many, a downward spiral of despair takes hold.

The Healing Challenge

Fortunately, that's right where *The Headache Healer's Handbook* comes in. This book walks you through the Mundo Program of mind-body therapies and practices to help you identify, reduce, and eliminate the causes of your headaches — and improve your overall health. It isn't magic; it's cause and effect: you make changes and get a new result.

By uncovering the clues in your daily life and understanding how they relate to your headaches, individually and in combination, you can crack the case like a detective. You will be successful if you are aware, thorough, and take each step slowly — and if you are willing to take new actions and shift old habits. After all, even a pill won't work if you don't swallow it. If you accept the challenge, your headaches will diminish and disappear.

Everything counts. Everything you do and are adds up to your pain. Change occurs when you claim self-empowerment, use "beginner's mind," incorporate stress reduction and hands-on therapies, and examine the deeper realms of your life. As the program unfolds, you will be able to summon your inner headache warrior, detective, and coach.

Somatic Self-Care

This self-care path takes a somatic approach, which means it works with your inner awareness of body, mind, emotions, and spirit. The term *somatics*, coined by Dr. Thomas Hanna, derives from the Greek word *soma*, or "living body." A somatic approach defines the body as an expression of one's entire being. More than simply a collection of mechanical parts, the body holds our life experience, including our history, and shapes our thinking, language, moods, and actions.

But how can somatic awareness heal headaches if modern medicine can't? Somatic self-care addresses a different realm than that of standard medical treatment and even some alternative therapies. In a somatic approach, the treatment *is* the process. It empowers you to take healing into your own hands. A pill doesn't address why and how you collect stress in your shoulders, clench your jaw, or stop breathing. Neither does it teach you how those factors contribute to your headaches, how to change them, or when and why you first embodied them.

Beyond tips and techniques, somatic self-care builds awareness of your automatic, unproductive reactions or patterns when they arise. It includes your inner experience and opens possibilities for shifting yourself in the moment. In this way, you can affect those seemingly unbreakable patterns that have added to your stress and challenged your health.

Life without Headaches: A Coach's Promise

How can you change your outlook from one of despair, fear, and powerlessness to one of faith, hope, and empowerment? With the help of a coach, of course!

A great coach, healer, teacher, or mentor in any domain is someone who believes in and sees the best in you. A coach tells you that you can and will do better and supports you in reaching your goals. A coach helps you look at things in new ways, kicks your butt if you lose your way, encourages you to get back on the horse when you fall off, and tells you to keep going when you want to give up. A coach keeps you focused on what is important and teaches you how to weigh your options and make choices based on your goals. A coach holds your big vision for you when you can't, don't, or won't and reminds you when you forget or forget how.

The Mundo Program is designed to be your personal headache coach. By taking on the practices and integrating the material in these pages, you will know more about yourself and your headaches, gain better health, and feel empowered to take charge of your life in many areas. In the process you will learn to rely on your own vision to see the big picture as well as the small one and to trust yourself to evaluate your options, make choices, and correct course if you falter. In the end, you will have become your own coach and healer.

For Kids and Teens Too

This book is for anyone who wants to both relieve and prevent headaches naturally, which includes kids and teens.

Some children and adolescents I've worked with started suffering from headaches as young as five and six years old — and some can't recall a time without them. Because their pain began at such tender ages, it's as if their bodies were readouts of the stress around them. Some felt tension or upheaval at home from divorce, illness, or familial birth or death; some were coping with bullying, trauma, or relocating to a new home, school, or city. Some were influenced by negative messages about diet, weight, appearance, and belonging. Some kids felt pressure to be perfect, excel, and win, while others felt frustrated and isolated because they were always sick with migraine. They carried the burden of their emotions (and often the result of "plain ole" bad habits) in their headaches.

Luckily, kids respond well to information about food, diet, and exercise, and are even open to learning new ways to calm down, like meditation or changes in their breathing and posture. Just as with adults, the key for kids is finding the right combination for each person, creating motivation, and teaching them *and* their parents. Instead of taking medications, they learn to make the connections between their stressors and their headaches, along with practical things they can do to avoid pain.

For Family and Friends: How to Help

Family and friends of people with migraine can feel helpless because they want to do something but don't know what to do or how to do it. If you are reading this book to support someone you care about, bravo!

Migraineurs are super sensitive to all stimuli, including touch, so it can be hard to know what is helpful or why your usually effective massage is not being welcomed. Not feeling well, migraine sufferers often withdraw from their usual family, work, and social activities, which can strain relationships and commitments — and then they feel bad or guilty about that too.

In these pages, you will find a variety of ways to help and support your family member or friend with migraine, and hopefully you will be inspired to add healthy living practices to your own life. Most people don't want to be treated differently because they are sick — especially children and teens. If the whole family has a healthy diet, your child, teenager, or spouse will feel that it's the norm. The same goes for postural awareness and stress reduction practices like breathing and meditation. By following the program, friends and family members can help while improving their own health.

It's true: some people have never experienced a migraine. If you have never had one and are trying to support someone who does, the first step is understanding how disabling it is. Try to recall the worst hangover you have ever had. If you are underage or have never had a hangover, do you remember having a fever, cold, virus, flu, infection, or other illness that left you feeling as sick as a dog, with your head about to explode?

In migraine, as with hangovers and illnesses, the symptoms are not just in your head, which would be bad enough. They take over your entire body. You feel overpowered, weak, and nauseated. Your skin turns pallid. The slightest movement makes you feel worse, and lights, sounds, and scents become magnified. You're disoriented and can't think straight, let alone sit or stand. You feel lucky to make it to the bathroom to throw up a few times, have the dry heaves with what's left, and make it back into bed.

You get the picture. Although everyone's experience is slightly different, if you have ever suffered like that, you have a glimpse into the world of migraine sufferers — except that their condition returns, often unpredictably, again and again. Can you see why someone would be sensitive to remarks like "How bad can it be — it's only a headache"? Your empathy and gentle suggestions can be more helpful than you realize.

Make Sure You're Okay, Then Proceed

The program and methods in these pages are not a substitute for medical advice. Before you proceed, make sure you have gotten a headache diagnosis from your doctor to rule out any other serious causes. All my headache clients are, or have been, under the care of neurologists and were initially examined by their primary care providers.

If you experience a negative change, especially a sudden worsening, in your regular headaches or headache patterns, whether or not you have had a diagnosis, contact your doctor right away!

Most headaches are *primary* and *inorganic*, which means that (1) the headache is the actual cause of the pain and (2) you can't locate it in a fixed, physical spot in your head, like a tumor, for example.

Secondary headache means that the headache is secondary to an underlying organic, often more serious condition, such as a concussion, brain tumor, cancer, meningitis, or an aneurysm.[5] If an underlying condition related to injury, illness, or disease is causing your headache, get treatment for it immediately.

If you are taking medication for your headaches, continue to work in conjunction with your doctor. After you have a strong grounding in mind-body practices for relief and prevention and your headaches have become less frequent and intense, you can ask the prescribing doctor for a regimen to help you stair-step down slowly from the medication you are taking.

How to Read This Book

Although you might be tempted to skip directly to the acute treatment parts of the book that show how to relieve your headache or migraine on the spot, don't do it! Transforming long-standing chronic headache patterns is a process that requires you to integrate new practices one by one, over time.

For example, I typically work with clients in fifteen to twenty one-hour weekly sessions, and more if we do bodywork or headache relief, or if a client has a history of trauma. A class series typically runs eight weeks, two hours per week. Both have homework and practices in between. The weekly spacing allows participants to integrate a new practice before learning the next, and I encourage you to take your time in working through the chapters.

The pacing depends on the individual because each person's

headache puzzle is different. Find what feels balanced for you. Some areas might take more of your attention than others. You have the book, and you always have your body, so you don't necessarily have to wait a whole week for each new lesson. The idea is to take action without getting overwhelmed. If you read through but don't engage, you will stand still. If you go too quickly (e.g., quitting caffeine cold turkey), you might get rebound headache. If you go too slowly, the continuity of balancing multiple life factors could get lost.

Here's what I recommend: To achieve the promised results, follow the program steps in order. Each practice teaches the skills needed to advance to the next level. That way, you will develop as you go, build on what you learn, and be prepared for each new step.

On the other hand, if you do have a headache or migraine episode (from a nonserious or previously diagnosed condition), you *might* try skipping to the hands-on therapies in part 4. Then, when you are feeling better, you can return to the prevention chapters about diet and stress reduction, which are vital components of the Mundo Program.

Like Rome, your headaches weren't built in a day, and they need to be carefully deconstructed brick by brick. As you build your new foundation, you will have all the tools you need to reassemble yourself into a healthier person. By embodying each new skill in turn, you will give yourself the best chance for success.

Your Support Team

Making lifestyle changes is no small feat, and it's helpful to have support. If you have a friend who has headaches, why not enlist each other as headache healing buddies? How about forming a group with several people, so you can read the book and implement the lessons, exercises, and practices together?

Whether you're reading this on your own or with a buddy or

group, the goal is to go beyond reading and move into action, which is the only thing that will change your situation. A support group, whether in-person or online, can provide a forum for sharing information — new books, therapies, and approaches — with people just like you who understand. But to make change, you must move beyond information and research. The headache healer's philosophy is proactive. It's not enough to read, plan, or hope; we have to *act* and institute new ways of being. To that end, a support group whose members encourage each other to make changes, stay on track, and leave their headaches behind can be very valuable.

Surround yourself with people who focus on positive change, committed listening, and taking action. Notice the mood and tone of the group you join. Do you leave feeling positive and energized? Is it rigorous and compassionate, or does it keep people stuck and complaining? Shaming or sentimentality can spiral downward into self-blame and victimhood — and a know-it-all who takes over and inserts opinions aggressively can stifle progress and make you doubt your own inner voice.

Look for avenues where you can give and receive strength and helpful encouragement to keep your momentum going. Put yourself out there instead of retreating and feeling misunderstood or ashamed. I encourage you to admit your truth and engage with others in a community of healing. It's a giant step forward.

2   What's Your Headache Type?

W hat's your type? No, not your blood type or the type of man or woman you are attracted to! I mean your headache type.

In this chapter, we examine the characteristics and symptoms of four basic headache types — *tension, migraine, cluster,* and *medication-overuse* headache — and describe danger signals of headaches that are caused by more serious medical conditions. We also look at the characteristics of headaches formerly known as *mixed* and now folded into the diagnosis of migraine. (As a reminder: This book is educational and does not diagnose, so please get a diagnosis from your healthcare provider.)

The International Classification of Headache Disorders, 3rd edition (the beta version, abbreviated here as ICHD-3 beta), defines and codes headache types so that doctors can diagnose and prescribe treatments for their patients.[1] Created by a committee of the International Headache Society, this diagnostic tool classifies headaches by characteristics, symptoms, and frequency into approximately three hundred types and subtypes, ranging from episodic to chronic and primary to secondary.

With a mind-body approach, we don't use the classifications for diagnosis and prescription. Instead, by knowing your headache type, you can demystify your symptoms and know which practices and therapies to turn to and when. Can you find your headache type below? Do any of the definitions fit your diagnosis or what you had suspected? Keep in mind that research and definitions evolve over time, and your symptoms may span several categories. As a neurologist specializing in headache noted — of course, all this was decided by a committee, and patients often don't fit into neat categories.

Types of Headaches

The following definitions include qualitative, somatic descriptions and ICHD-3 beta classification parameters.

Tension-Type Headache

Popularly known as *tension headache*, tension-type headache is the most common and least-researched headache type. It is characterized by tightness and pressure on both sides of the head, and the pain, which is steady, dull, and nonpulsating, is compared to a tight hatband or having one's head stuck in a vise. People often complain of a stuck, knot-like pain in the lower skull, back of the neck, shoulders, upper back, or jaw. Tension headache was previously termed *muscle contraction headache* because those areas can feel tender, tight, and contracted. Tension headache can last from thirty minutes to a week.

Routine physical activity does not tend to make these headaches worse, nor are they accompanied by nausea or vomiting, as in migraine. Nevertheless, they can be debilitating. Some people with tension headache are sensitive to light or sound. If tension headache occurs fifteen or more days per month for three months or more and is not due to medication overuse, the diagnosis changes from *episodic* to *chronic* tension-type headache.

Migraine

Migraine is a primary disorder that is characterized by recurrent, debilitating attacks of throbbing, pulsing, or pounding pain, usually located at the sides and front of the head and face, especially forehead and temples. Despite its origins in the Latin term *hemicrania* — meaning "half skull," because the pain is often one-sided — migraine can affect one or both sides of the head. During an episode, the pain can even move around — or migrate from one side to the other. An episode typically lasts four to seventy-two hours and is often accompanied by other symptoms.

Migraine is divided into two main subtypes. *Migraine without aura* (previously termed *common migraine*) is the most common. *Migraine with aura*, previously termed *classic migraine*, is preceded or accompanied by a set of neurological symptoms, collectively termed *aura*, that can last from several minutes to an hour. Visual disturbances are the most common aura type and can take the form of scintillations — such as flickering lights, spots, or lines — and scotoma, a loss of some or all of a visual field that is otherwise normal. Other types of auras are described as pins and needles on one side of the body or face, numbness, and speech disturbances. Aura symptoms are completely reversible but can be alarming, especially before you are diagnosed, because they are so unusual.

Additionally, migraine can have *premonitory symptoms* (also called the *prodrome phase*) that occur two to forty-eight hours before an episode. These symptoms include neck stiffness; sensitivity to light, sound, and odors; fatigue; elation; depression; unusual hunger; particular food cravings; yawning; and pallor.

Symptoms can also manifest during the resolution or recovery phase of the migraine. Although this phase, called the *postdrome*, is not included in the ICHD-3 beta, many patients report a distinct phase following their migraines. It can last from six to twenty-four hours and has nonheadache symptoms similar to those of the other phases, including most frequently fatigue and neck pain, also light, sound, and odor sensitivities, disorientation, and appetite loss.[2]

Two important subtypes of migraine are *menstrual migraine*, which occurs just before or at the beginning of the menstrual cycle, and *menstrual-related migraine*, which presents at other times during the month in addition to the menstrual migraine pattern.[3] (There's more about migraine and hormones in chapter 8.)

Migraine sufferers seek the stimulus-free environment of a dark, quiet room. They are sensitive to light, odors, sound, and touch; and they have visual field disturbances and mood changes. Even the slightest movement can set off a wave of associated symptoms, including nausea and vomiting. These symptoms can feel just as debilitating as the head pain.

When complicated by other factors, such as muscle tension or medication overuse, a migraine can last for weeks or months, turning it into a chronic condition. Migraine is diagnosed as *chronic* when episodes occur more than fifteen days per month over a period of three months, provided they are not caused by medication overuse.

Headaches Formerly Known as Mixed

Many people get symptoms of tension headache along with their migraine. This headache type was previously termed *coexisting migraine and tension-type headache* and prior to that was known as *the mixed headache syndrome*.

In ICHD-3 beta, this combination of symptoms is no longer classified as a distinct headache type; instead, the symptoms associated with tension-type headache are folded into the diagnosis of chronic migraine. These headaches often begin in tight, painful points or contracted areas in the lower skull, neck, shoulders, or upper back (commonly in the same spot each time). The pain migrates to the entire head or to specific areas in the forehead, temples, and face, where it escalates into pulsing, pounding pain, accompanied by nausea, vomiting, and other migraine symptoms.

Medication-Overuse Headache

Medication-overuse headache (MOH) is caused by regular and extended use of medication — whether prescription, nonprescription, or a combination of both. It is diagnosed when a headache is present on fifteen or more days per month. These headaches can be caused by taking one or more acute or symptomatic treatment drugs ten times per month, or about two days per week, for three months.

This headache type is considered secondary because it is caused by something more — in this case, use of medication. Formerly called *rebound, drug-induced,* or *medication-misuse headache,* this condition has become so common, due to the growing preponderance of medications taken to treat headache and migraine, that these diagnostic categories were created in response.

In addition to headache frequency, diagnosis of MOH is determined by the class of medication that is being overused, including ergotamine, triptan, analgesic, opioid, a combination of acute-use medications or analgesics, and other medication not specifically taken for headache. Pain-relief preparations that combine analgesics, barbiturates, or opioids with caffeine are designed for short-term use, and if overused or taken over time, they can transform episodic, occasional migraine into a chronic condition.

Cluster Headache

Known as the most painful primary headache, cluster headache is most prevalent in men and is the least common type. Its name refers to the frequency of attacks, which occur in clusters of time. Episodes often persist for weeks or months, disappear for months or years, then reappear. Each attack can last from fifteen minutes to three hours, and attacks can occur up to eight times per day, although less frequent occurrence, such as every other day, is also common. Patients tend to have episodes during the same season or month each year, so there has been speculation that cluster headaches are linked to circadian rhythms. The published clinical research by Lee Kudrow, Sr., MD, showed the positive results of oxygen therapy,[4] which makes me wonder if breathing exercises could provide relief.

Cluster headache pain and its unique symptoms are different from those of migraine and characterized by sharp, stabbing pain in one eye, with watering of the same-side nostril. Patients become agitated and are known to pace the floor and bang their heads against the wall for relief. (Contrast that with migraine sufferers, who must lie down in darkened rooms and remain still.) Cluster headache pain is so relentlessly intense that it has been linked to incidence of suicide, resulting in the nickname "suicide headache." Extremely painful headaches of other types can be mistakenly diagnosed as cluster headaches, even though the symptoms might not fit.

Because very few clients in my practice have had a diagnosis of cluster headache, this book does not devote special attention to it. Among that group, those who reported combined symptoms of tension, migraine, and cluster headache — neck pain, nausea, throbbing, and stabbing in one eye — were able to overcome them by completing the program.

When Headache Is a Danger Sign

If you are experiencing a sudden-onset headache with severe, constant pain — the worst ever — or a recurrence and worsening of an intensely painful headache or migraine, it can be a sign of something more serious, such as an infection, meningitis, a virus, flu, concussion, brain tumor, or brain aneurysm. Migraine can signal life-threatening complications during and following birth, including preeclampsia, eclampsia, thrombosis, and brain hemorrhage.

If you have unusual symptoms along with your headache, including fever, dizziness, drowsiness, weakness, numbness, chills, or loss of balance, contact your doctor right away. Was this particular headache brought on or made worse by exertion, sexual activity, coughing, or straining? Pay attention to these signals, especially if your first headache strikes when you are forty or older.

Is it the worst headache of your life? Even with a previous diagnosis, this symptom can signal that your headache is a secondary symptom of a serious health condition that needs immediate medical attention. Especially if your headache is sudden and different, it is always wise to err on the side of caution. Whether you already have a diagnosis or not, if you have any of the above symptoms, immediately contact your doctor or go to the emergency room!

Headache or Migraine?

A lot of the information in this book applies to tension-type headache, migraine, and combinations thereof. So for brevity's sake, I often use the word *headache* to include them all, without naming each one. Of course, they are different, and I would never confuse or conflate them — nor would I minimize a migraine by calling it "only a headache."

Rest assured that when a specific therapy, practice, or technique is meant for a particular headache type, especially in the case of migraine, I will make that distinction. For example, some people can relieve their tension headaches by exercising, but that would be a horrible remedy for someone in the midst of a migraine who can barely move, much less exercise.

3   Your Personal Headache Profile

*L*et's add the most important ingredient: you!

Starting on the next page, you will fill out the Headache History Questionnaire and record information about your typical headaches, possible triggers, food and exercise habits, medication use, significant life events, and more. Your responses will form your baseline and will be used again at the end of the program to evaluate your progress.

The headache history questions are designed not only to provide baseline information but to help you begin the inquiry process of looking at your headaches in a new light. Some questions might awaken memories and reveal decisions made long ago that impact you today. Be open, and let the process spark your curiosity and provide new clues. By examining the details and aspects of your life in order to discover their connections, you are embarking on the foundational practice of the headache healer.

Headache History Questionnaire

Complete the questionnaire. Use separate or additional paper if you wish.

1. Date: _____

2. Name: _____

3. Status (circle): Single Married Partnered Divorced Widowed

4. Children's names/ages: _____
   _____

5. Occupation: _____

6. a. Number of years at your work or job: _____
   b. Do you like your work? yes _____ no _____

7. a. Age now: _____   b. Age at onset: _____
   c. Number of years with headaches: _____

8. a. Height: _____   b. Weight: _____

9. Circle the type(s) of headaches you have:

   tension-type headache
   migraine without aura
   migraine with aura
   migraine with symptoms of tension-type headache
   tension-type headache with symptoms of migraine
   menstrual migraine
   menstrual-related migraine
   medication-overuse headache
   cluster headache

10. Describe where your headache pain is usually located: _____
    _____

11. How often do you get headaches?
    # per week: _____ or # per month: _____ or # per year: _____

12. How long do your headaches usually last?
    # of minutes: _____ or # of hours: _____ or # of days: _____

13. Circle all symptoms you get *before* a migraine, during the premonitory phase / prodrome:

anxiety	head pain	smell sensitivity
constipation	hyperactivity	sound sensitivity
depression	insomnia	stuffy nose
diarrhea	light sensitivity	touch/skin sensitivity
disorientation	loss of appetite	(allodynia)
dizziness	mood changes	visual changes
face pain	nausea	visual distortion
fatigue	neck pain	vomiting
frequent urination	shoulder pain	yawning
hallucinations		

    other (describe): _____

14. How long before your headaches start do these symptoms typically occur? _____

15. If you have migraine with aura, describe your aura symptoms:

    _____

16. Circle the word(s) that best describe your typical headache pain:

aching	intermittent	sore
band-like	painful	stabbing
beating	piercing	stake-like
boring	poking	steady
constant	pounding	tender
drilling	pulsating	throbbing
dull	sharp	tight
gripping	shooting	viselike
hurting		

17. Indicate the usual intensity of your headaches by circling a number on the pain scale:

    0   1   2   3   4   5   6   7   8   9   10

    No pain   Most intense
                                                     pain imaginable

18. Circle other symptoms you get *during* a headache:

anxiety	general pain	sinus pain
appetite loss	hallucinations	smell sensitivity
back pain	lethargy	soreness
constipation	light sensitivity	sound sensitivity
depression	mood changes	tenderness
diarrhea	nausea	touch/skin sensitivity
dizziness	neck pain	(allodynia)
face pain	scalp pain	visual changes
fatigue	shoulder pain	vomiting

other (describe): _____

19. Do you wake up with headaches? yes _____ no _____

20. Circle any factors that seem to trigger your headaches:

Dietary
aged cheeses
alcohol/alcoholic
   beverages
artificial sweeteners
beans
beer
caffeine
chocolate
citrus fruits
dairy products
fatty foods
food sensitivity
   (list): _____
   _____
hot dogs
irregular eating
lack of caffeine
lack of water
low blood sugar
luncheon meats
MSG
nitrates, nitrites
nuts
pickled foods
preservatives, chemi-
   cal additives
skipping meals
sugar
wheat gluten
wine, red
wine, white

Hormonal
birth
birth control (pills,
   IUD, patch)
hormone replace-
   ment therapy
menarche (onset of
   first period)
menopause
menstruation
ovulation
perimenopause
pregnancy

Environmental
air pollution
bright light
chemical sensitivity
cigarette smoke
cold
damp weather
dim light
dry air
fluorescent lighting
fumes
heat
high altitude
hot, dry winds
humidity
loud noise
low barometric
   pressure
perfume, scents
stormy weather
strong odors
sun overexposure
weather changes

Lifestyle	Medication	Physical
cigarette smoking	analgesic, simple (overuse)	allergy
disrupted sleep		cell phone (texting), electronic device use
excessive sleep	analgesic, combination (overuse)	
fatigue		computer overuse
insufficient sleep	antiasthma drugs	exercise
let-down headache	antidepressants	exertion from sex
motion	antiseizure drugs	exertion from sports
recreational drugs	blood pressure drugs	eyestrain
routine change	blood vessel dilators	flu, cold, or virus
stress	diuretics	head trauma
travel	"drug cocktail" (combining several medications)	neck, shoulder, back tension
		poor posture
	ergotamine overuse	sedentary lifestyle
	opioid overuse	sinusitis, rhinitis
	triptan overuse	

anything else (in any category): _____

21. How many hours of quality sleep do you get per night? _____

22. How much of the following do you drink daily?
    water (# oz.): _____ coffee (# oz.): _____ tea (# oz.): _____
    espresso (# shots): _____ cola (# oz.): _____ soda (# oz.): _____

23. List the approximate times of day you eat:
    breakfast: _____ AM snack: _____ AM lunch: _____ PM
    snack: _____ PM dinner: _____ PM snack: _____ PM

24. List what you typically eat for each meal and snack:
    Breakfast: _____
    Morning snack: _____
    Lunch: _____
    Afternoon snack: _____
    Dinner: _____
    Evening snack: _____

25. Do you exercise? yes _____ no _____
    If yes, how many times per week? _____
    How many minutes per session? _____
    Type(s) of exercise: _____

26. Circle the types of practitioner you have seen for your headaches:

acupuncturist/DOM	herbalist	osteopath
allergist	homeopath	pain specialist
bodyworker	massage therapist	physical therapist
chiropractor	naturopath	primary care provider
craniosacral therapist	neurologist	psychiatrist
dentist	nurse practitioner	psychologist
ENT (ear, nose, and	OB/GYN	registered dietitian,
throat doctor; or	occupational therapist	nutritionist
otolaryngologist)	ophthalmologist	Reiki or energy-work
general practitioner	optometrist	practitioner
healer	orthodontist	social worker

    other (describe): _____

27. List headache medications taken during the past five years (prescription and over-the-counter):

MEDICATION: _____

Dose unit (tablet/tsp/mg/ml): _____ Frequency (per day/week/month): _____

Dates taken: _____ to _____   # of years taken: _____   Still use? ❑ yes ❑ no

Effective? ❑ yes ❑ no   Side effects? ❑ yes ❑ no

List side effects: _____

Reason(s) stopped or still using: _____

MEDICATION: _____

Dose unit (tablet/tsp/mg/ml): _____ Frequency (per day/week/month): _____

Dates taken: _____ to _____   # of years taken: _____   Still use? ❑ yes ❑ no

Effective? ❑ yes ❑ no   Side effects? ❑ yes ❑ no

List side effects: _____

Reason(s) stopped or still using: _____

MEDICATION: _____

Dose unit (tablet/tsp/mg/ml): _____ Frequency (per day/week/month): _____

Dates taken: ____ to ____   # of years taken: ____   Still use? ❑ yes ❑ no

Effective? ❑ yes ❑ no   Side effects? ❑ yes ❑ no

List side effects: _____

Reason(s) stopped or still using: _____

28. List other medications taken regularly over the past five years (for example, medication for birth control, hormone replacement, thyroid condition, blood pressure, heart condition, chronic pain, depression, sleep issues, anxiety, or sinus condition):

MEDICATION: _____

Dose unit (tablet/tsp/mg/ml): _____ Frequency (per day/week/month): _____

Dates taken: ____ to ____   # of years taken: ____   Still use? ❑ yes ❑ no

Effective? ❑ yes ❑ no   Side effects? ❑ yes ❑ no

List side effects: _____

Reason(s) stopped or still using: _____

MEDICATION: _____

Dose unit (tablet/tsp/mg/ml): _____ Frequency (per day/week/month): _____

Dates taken: ____ to ____   # of years taken: ____   Still use? ❑ yes ❑ no

Effective? ❑ yes ❑ no   Side effects? ❑ yes ❑ no

List side effects: _____

Reason(s) stopped or still using: _____

MEDICATION: _____

Dose unit (tablet/tsp/mg/ml): _____ Frequency (per day/week/month): _____

Dates taken: ____ to ____   # of years taken: ____   Still use? ❑ yes ❑ no

Effective? ❑ yes ❑ no   Side effects? ❑ yes ❑ no

List side effects: _____

Reason(s) stopped or still using: _____

29. Circle any other therapies you have tried for your headaches:

Therapy	Currently using?		Effective?		
	Yes	No	Yes	No	Not sure
Acupuncture	❏	❏	❏	❏	❏
Biofeedback	❏	❏	❏	❏	❏
Bodywork	❏	❏	❏	❏	❏
Breathing	❏	❏	❏	❏	❏
Cannabis	❏	❏	❏	❏	❏
Chiropractic	❏	❏	❏	❏	❏
Cold pack	❏	❏	❏	❏	❏
Diet (special)	❏	❏	❏	❏	❏
Exercise	❏	❏	❏	❏	❏
Herbs	❏	❏	❏	❏	❏
Hot pack	❏	❏	❏	❏	❏
Massage	❏	❏	❏	❏	❏
Meditation	❏	❏	❏	❏	❏
Relaxation	❏	❏	❏	❏	❏
Shower/bath	❏	❏	❏	❏	❏
Sleep/rest	❏	❏	❏	❏	❏
Stretching	❏	❏	❏	❏	❏
Supplements	❏	❏	❏	❏	❏
Vitamins	❏	❏	❏	❏	❏
Yoga	❏	❏	❏	❏	❏
other: _____	❏	❏	❏	❏	❏

30. Do you have any hobbies? If so, please list them:

31. Describe any traumas, illnesses, or significant life events, including any that occurred during your perinatal and early life.

32. What was going on in your life when your headaches first began?

33. What do you think causes your headaches, based on what you know so far?

34. What is stressful or causes stress in your life?

35. Do you have any other health concerns? If so, please describe.

36. Is anything missing from your life that you would like to have in it?

37. Imagine your life as free of headaches. Describe what that would be and look like, and how it would be different from your current life.

38. Write anything else you would like to express about yourself, your family, your headaches, or your life.

Your Observations

Now that you have recorded the details of your history and daily life, did this process stir the pot or remind you of things you had forgotten? Your recollections are the perfect place to start mining your life for clues. I'll illustrate my point using four of the questions you've answered as examples.

Questions 5 and 6, about occupation, seems pretty straightforward at first. But if you think about all the factors involved in your work and how you use your body throughout your day, there might be more to that seemingly simple question.

What does your occupation have to do with your headaches? Let's explore:

- Notice whether you sit at your desk or computer in the same position or perform repetitive tasks for hours at a time without moving, getting up, taking breaks, or eating lunch. Is your head typically pulled forward toward your computer? Is your neck bent while you text? Is your body often torqued — for example as you reach sideways for items on your desk?

- Think about your posture and the stress you experience as you commute, drive for your job, or chauffeur your kids around. Notice whether your lower back is supported, whether your shoulders are relaxed or raised up, and how tightly you are gripping the wheel. If you walk or bike to work, consider the weight of your bag, backpack, or briefcase over one or both shoulders.

- Consider your workplace, whether it's outside of or in your home, and whether it is a stressful place. What is your mood about it? Perhaps you are responsible for other people — employees, clients, patients, or customers — for their livelihoods, or even their lives. Perhaps you like your occupation but dislike your workplace or some of your coworkers and would rather be working somewhere else. Perhaps you are unemployed and desperately need a job. Does the stress of your workplace affect your emotional health? Your physical health?

If you have aches and pains at the end of the day, any of the above factors, and more, connected with your work or your job could be causing them. Consider the tangible and intangible factors involved in doing your job and balancing your work with the rest of your life.

Next let's touch on questions 31 and 32, which ask about your life when your headaches first began. Reflect on that time and how what was happening affected your body, your self, and your sense of safety:

- Were you injured or ill, or did you have an accident? Were you going through a difficult personal or family situation? Did you move to a new area or change schools? Were you traumatized, assaulted, or abused?
- Perhaps you were going through hormonal changes, or starting contraceptives, hormone replacement therapy, or new medication.
- If you were starting college and living away from home for the first time, think about your newfound freedoms; any academic, athletic, or social pressures; and the changes in your eating, drinking, sleeping, and postural habits.
- If you were an adult, think of all you were trying to juggle between spouse, kids, and work — or any job or financial uncertainty.

You can mine all of your answers for clues in this way. Some questions might seem more relevant to you than others, but any of them could reveal triggers you might have previously discounted, like starting or stopping a medication, hobby, job, or routine. So consider everything, and don't give anything short shrift. The hidden gems are often found where you least expect them, and others could bubble up later.

The Power of Your Story

Your story has power. Each chronic headache sufferer has a story, and telling yours — describing the pain and giving voice to the frustration you've experienced in trying to heal it — brings its power to the fore. Part of the healing journey is learning how to spot clues in order to gain insight, and both clues and insight might be hidden in your story. This section introduces you to a new way of listening to your inner voice — a practice that continues throughout the healing process.

Early on in my practice, as I led classes of patients who were referred by their neurologists, we would do brief introductions on the first day and check-ins throughout the course. The depth of pain and suffering and the mood in which each person told his or her story spoke volumes.

> Hi, my name is Carol. I've had migraines for thirty years now, since I was fourteen. I get them every day, and I've been using over-the-counter pain medication daily for the past ten years. I'm afraid that if I stop taking it, the pain will be even worse. My headache doctor referred me to this class, and I'm skeptical of trying one more thing. But I'm here to give it a shot.

Based on my somatics training, I would listen to each story by centering in my body and holding a neutral space. By *neutral space*, I mean a feeling of empathy for the person without falling into sentimentality about their pain. (More "I hear you" and less "Oh, you poor dear, that's horrible.") While holding a vision for each person's healing, I could also hear voice quality and tone, word choices, mood, and posture — which would inform my assessments and coaching. To my surprise, the classes spontaneously adopted my mode of listening, and whoever was sharing would start to listen to herself in that way too. It was so touching to feel that mood of compassion pervade the room.

Finding a setting in which you can tell your story and listen to the stories of others can be revealing and helpful. Although it can be hard to imagine beforehand, there is usually someone who is worse off than you are, and hearing their story lets you empathize and takes the focus off your own pain. ("Geez, and I thought that *I* had it bad.") Hearing someone in the group talk about doing better shows you that the possibility for healing exists. ("If *she*'s doing better, maybe there's hope for *me*.") And, of course, being heard and believed is internally settling.

The story you tell yourself and others about your headaches plays a powerful role in healing them. Listen to the words and the voice you use to describe your pain, yourself, and your life. Try to listen to yourself and others with compassion — as if you were in that classroom of headache patients, hearing their headache stories and being heard.

4 The Mind-Body-Headache Connection

In his writings, seventeenth-century French philosopher René Descartes assigned the flesh and blood of humans to medicine and their spiritual side to the church, and it stuck. In Western culture, we tend to move through life as if our bodies are simply vehicles on which to carry our heads around — just well-oiled machines unrelated to our thoughts, aspirations, and behaviors.

In the 1960s, Eastern spiritual philosophies and practices began flooding into Western culture. Over the next forty years, a large variety of meditation, yoga, tai chi, martial arts, and bodywork disciplines became widely available, and new forms were created and adopted. Classes were offered at medical centers and sports clubs; doctors referred patients to complementary medicine practitioners; and the National Institutes of Health (NIH) began researching alternative therapies in medicine. People who practiced these disciplines and received these therapies found that relaxing their bodies calmed their minds, and calming their minds relaxed their bodies.

What Is the Mind-Body Connection?

The term *mind-body* (or *body-mind*) is used in conjunction with health and healing. For nearly a century, researchers have been trying to prove what Eastern and indigenous cultures have known and practiced for millennia (and what Descartes had wrong): People are more than their flesh and blood. Rather than being purely mechanical operating systems, living beings have intuitive intelligence, from the cellular to the cosmic level.

The mind-body connection means that your body and mind are one; they are inextricably connected and constantly interacting. But what *is* this connection, why is it significant, and what does it have to do with headaches?

The Biofeedback Revolution

At about the same time mind-body approaches were growing in popularity, biofeedback therapy created a revolution in the scientific world when it showed that people could exert voluntary control over their own nervous system functions that were previously thought to be involuntary. The *central nervous system*, made of the brain and spinal cord, sends and receives information to and from the body via the *peripheral nervous system*, which has two branches: (1) The *somatic nervous system* controls conscious, voluntary functions, like skeletal and muscular systems, and general senses, like pain, temperature, touch, vision, hearing, and joint position. (2) The *autonomic nervous system* controls unconscious, involuntary actions — like heart rate, respiration, skin temperature, blood flow, and digestion — and cardiac and smooth muscle (blood vessel) tissue.[1]

The two branches of the autonomic nervous system govern the body at rest and in action: (1) the *parasympathetic nervous system* (PNS), which is the body in balance, or *homeostasis*, governs the body at rest, and (2) the *sympathetic nervous system* (SNS), which mobilizes the fight-or-flight response, governs the body during activity.

In biofeedback training, a patient, who is fitted with sensors and hooked up to an electronic device, learns relaxation techniques, then receives instant feedback of the results through the device via sound or visual cues. Researchers showed that trainees could engage their PNS, slowing heart rate and respiration and aiding digestion, and override their SNS. The goal of the training is to reproduce those relaxed states using mind-body cues in lieu of the device's feedback.

Biofeedback Pioneers

In the 1930s, German psychiatrist Johannes Heinrich Schultz developed autogenic training, where people are taught to use mental visualizations, passive concentration, and verbal commands to induce a relaxation response ("Now my hands are heavy and warm"). In 1958, psychologist Joe Kamiya, PhD, experimented with electroencephalography (EEG), or brain-wave biofeedback, now known as *neurofeedback*, at the University of Chicago. Dr. Kamiya demonstrated that test subjects could learn to recognize when they were in relaxed, intuitive, alert mental states, called *alpha*, and control their brain waves to produce these states.[2]

In the 1970s, Joseph Sargent, Elmer Green, and Dale Walters of the Menninger Foundation began investigating the use of autogenic feedback training to control migraine and tension headache. By combining autogenic training and biofeedback, subjects were able to control heart rate, blood pressure, and extremities temperature.[3]

More research followed: In 1976, researchers Jose Medina, Seymour Diamond, and Mary Franklin showed that with skin-temperature and electromyographic biofeedback training, or EMG biofeedback, headache severity and frequency as well as medication usage decreased significantly.[4] Turin found that finger-temperature warming alone was effective in reducing migraine activity;[5] Sargent's study showed nondrug treatments for migraine decreased headache frequency;[6] and Mitchell and Mitchell combined relaxation, awareness, assertiveness, and desensitization trainings, resulting in markedly reduced headache frequency.[7]

Collectively, the research shows that you can learn to change your stress, tension, headaches, and pain with your mind.

Passive and Active Volition

Interestingly, biofeedback therapy makes a distinction between two mental states of volition, or exerting the will. In biofeedback, the patient does not attempt to actively will a state of homeostasis and calmness, which is called *active volition* ("I must relax!"). Instead, the patient produces relaxation using *passive volition*, which is an open and allowing awareness of one's inner world.[8]

Always versus Never

The most effective way to understand the mind-body connection and how it relates to your headaches is to experience it firsthand.

"Always versus Never" is an exercise I've adapted from the work of Clyde W. Ford, DC,[9] to demonstrate your mind-body connection in real time. It is based on working with two sets of thoughts, or inner dialogues. In my adaptation, each dialogue represents a way of thinking about your headaches — one negative, and one positive.

To do this exercise, first follow the setup instructions. Then read the scripts, do the exercise, and at the end do the check-in and debriefing.

If you are reading this book to support someone else, you can do the exercise too. Simply use a concern from any area of your life for your inner dialogue. Find something that is real for you right now and substitute your concern for the words *headaches*, *migraines*, or *pain* in the scripts.

Setup

First, stand in an area with enough space around you to extend your arms to the front, sides, back, and above your head. Then give yourself a good base: Place your feet hip-distance apart (about twelve inches) with your feet parallel, toes pointed forward or turned slightly in, knees soft and unlocked. This will give you good balance as you do the exercise with your eyes closed.

Scripts

Now read over the following two scripts of internal dialogue to familiarize yourself with them. During the actual exercise, your eyes will be closed as you repeat in your mind each set of thoughts. Don't worry about memorizing all the words — it's the thought that counts!

The first set of thoughts is called "Always":

SCRIPT 1: ALWAYS

"I'm *always* going to have these headaches (or these migraines). I'm *always* going to have this pain. I'm *always* going to feel sick. I thought this program would give me the answers, but now I have doubts. It's just another dead end. I feel lousy. I'm afraid I'll *always* be stuck here. There's no way out. No matter what I do, nothing ever changes; it's *always* the same. I hate this pain!"

Got that? Good. I know it can be hard to go there!

Now, read over the second set of thoughts, called "Never":

SCRIPT 2: NEVER

"I will *never* again have these headaches (or these migraines)! I will *never* again have this pain and disability. I will *not* suffer like this again. I've finally found the answers I've been looking for, and I'm *never* turning back. I feel so much better now. I see more possibilities. After all this time, I'm actually hopeful. I can live my life free of pain. I feel great! Yay! I'm free!"

Move to Match the Thought

Now that you know the thought scripts, it's time to add the special sauce. During the exercise, while you're saying each thought in your mind, *move your body to match the thought.* In whatever way feels right, allow your body to move in a way that expresses what you are thinking.

For example, when you say to yourself you'll always be in pain, do you tighten your shoulders and lower your head? What does your body do when you say you'll *never* be in pain? Whatever feels right for you, move to express each thought.

Always versus Never Exercise

Now read over the numbered steps that follow, glance at the scripts one more time if needed, and then put the book down. When you are ready to begin the exercise, return to your stance with feet hip-distance apart and knees soft, close your eyes, and proceed. When you finish the exercise, open your eyes and do the check-in and debriefing.

1. For about thirty seconds, repeat in your mind the "Always" script, or your version of "I am *always* going to have these headaches (or migraines). I am *always* going to be in pain. I am *always* going to have to curb my activities," and all the negative thoughts that go with it. Allow your body to move to match the thought "I *always* will have this pain."

2. Then switch to the "Never" script and repeat it in your mind for thirty seconds: "I am *never* again going to have these headaches (or migraines). I feel so much better! I am free!

Yay!" and all the positive thoughts that go with it. Allow your body to move to match and express the thought of "*Never again* will I have this pain."

3. When you're done, open your eyes, sit down, and do the check-in and debriefing that follows.

Check-In and Debriefing

1. What happened in your body during the exercise when thinking you would *always* have headaches, migraines, and pain?

    - What happened to your tension or relaxation overall? In specific areas?
    - What happened with your posture and breathing? How about your mood?

2. What happened to your body, posture, breathing, mood, tension, and relaxation when you thought you would *never again* have headaches, migraines, and pain?

3. Were your two responses different?

    - For *always*, did your body contract, shoulders raise, neck stiffen, and head pull in? Did you hold your breath? Was your mood fearful, hopeless, angry, sad?
    - For *never*, what happened? Did you feel a sense of relief, take a breath, let out a sigh, or smile? Could you let your body go, lift your head, and see beyond your pain? How did that feel?

You might have had the responses listed here, or others. During the Always exercise, some people grip their temples as if in pain, whereas others get completely still and don't want to move at all. Some follow their urge to self-soothe and simply hug themselves while standing, while others curl up in a fetal position. And while imagining being free from pain, some people extend their arms in the air in joy!

You might not have had the responses you expected. Some headache sufferers report they simply "can't go there" — meaning, they can't imagine *always* having pain — for fear of actually bringing on a headache. On the flipside, even *never* can be difficult for those who cannot imagine their world as pain-free. They are unable to get there mentally for fear of being disappointed again.

There are no right or wrong reactions, only what happens to you. Your palpable, felt responses — whether positive, negative, or reluctant — are what matter. It's okay if your responses are so subtle that an outside observer couldn't tell anything was happening. What matters is that *you* feel something happen and are aware of it.

Survival and Wonder Vision

We now return to the point of the Always versus Never exercise: to have an experience of your mind-body connection and understand how it relates to your headaches.

In the exercise, you spent a minute or so working with two types of thoughts, and you likely noticed that something happened in your body as a result. Did you contract or feel fear with the negative and expand and feel joy with the positive?

Of course, the directions were to move your body to match your thoughts. But I'm pretty sure that you didn't take a deep breath, lift your head, and raise your arms to the sky when imagining yourself stuck in pain — or tighten your body when imagining that you were free of it. We naturally contract when under stress and expand when feeling safe.

Here's the point. Your body responded to two types of thoughts in the period of just a minute. How many thoughts do you have in ten minutes, a half-hour, an hour, a day, a week? A lot! And your body is reacting to each one.

In fact, every thought has a bodily response. I repeat: there is no thinking without your body responding. If you are thinking angry or hopeless thoughts, what happens to your shoulders, jaw, posture, and mood? Your body responds. Every thought — happy, sad, angry, fearful, hopeful — has the potential to affect your headaches because it's affecting your body.

Body-centered psychotherapists Gay and Kathlyn Hendricks say that people view the world with either *survival vision* or *wonder vision*.[10] In survival mode we see the world through fear-tinted glasses, and those filters limit our choices. We feel like we're struggling tooth and nail just to make it. However, in wonder mode, we see the world through curiosity-tinted glasses. We allow ourselves to wonder about a problem and consider possible solutions instead of worrying about it.

Drawing from the Always versus Never exercise, thinking that you will always be in pain is like seeing the world with survival vision. It looks like there's no hope — your possibilities are limited and you're barely scraping by. In contrast, thinking that you can be over your headaches is like viewing the world with wonder vision. You can be hopeful and see a future filled with possibilities.

From Expert to Beginner

Why is it important to be open to new possibilities? By the time I meet my clients, most of them have tried many therapies and are skeptical after repeatedly chasing hope that ends in defeat. They have become experts at knowing what does or doesn't work for them, but they can be closed to exploring new avenues. They think they've already tried everything, and they don't want to put out the effort and risk more pain and disappointment. They've tried alternative therapies and wonder how somatic self-care is different.

In his classic book *Zen Mind, Beginner's Mind*, Zen master Shunryu Suzuki Roshi writes, "In the beginner's mind there are many possibilities, but in the expert's there are few."[11] Zen philosophy teaches us to live life in each moment — savoring, appreciating, and learning from it. That's beginner's mind. Having beginner's mind is like having wonder vision. Like a new puppy or kitten, we are open, inquisitive, and unjaded, and we want to explore everything. Beginner's mind is that willingness to begin again and again.

The first step in the Mundo Program is being willing to enter into a new inquiry process with fresh eyes despite what you have already tried. You might discover something that you missed previously — which is, after all, why we get second opinions about our health, our fashion choices, or anything else.

This process of looking at your headaches in new and different ways is more than a one-time exercise. You have to keep refreshing your vision if you get stuck and can't find answers. If you're in a negative mood and feel as if nothing is working, if you're questioning why you're putting yourself through this again, that means you're squarely in survival mode. It's time to re-up, find your bearings, move forward, and return to wonder mode. To do so, stop, acknowledge your mood, take a breath, and find center.

In chapters 11 and 12 you will learn meditation and breathing practices to help you to feel more calm and open.

Becoming a Headache Detective

Why do we love the image of a detective? Because detectives are dedicated to the case and intent on solving the mystery at hand. Using their wits, curiosity, and perseverance, they uncover clues and reveal possibilities that ultimately lead them to the culprit.

The beloved fictional detectives Sherlock Holmes and Lieutenant Columbo embody the energetic perseverance that is needed to crack difficult cases. They're the epitome of living in wonder mode — always poking and prodding what is hidden and what is obvious, plumbing the depths of the mystery, and searching for clues, for "just one more thing."

If you wanted a detective to solve your headache mystery, whom would you hire? If a detective said, "You know, I'm not sure I can help you. I've seen cases like yours before, and I'm not hopeful. But I can take your case anyway and see what I can do," would you hire that person? Me, I would turn around and walk away; I wouldn't even consider hiring someone who wasn't hopeful, open, and gung ho about my case.

I would want to hire the detective who greeted me with this:

> After you made your appointment, I did some initial legwork, and I've identified four doors worth exploring. In fact, I looked behind one of them, found a hallway, followed it to the end, found two more doors, looked behind each of them, found several clues, came back out, and am ready to explore what's behind the three other doors. What do you think?

When it comes to hiring the best person to solve your headaches, that detective is you! Be the detective you'd want to hire.

Placebo: Your Inner Warrior

The state of inner knowing and confidence, the belief that you can do something, is palpable in wonder mode. The power of belief is so real that it has a name in medical research: the *placebo effect*. The placebo effect is a beneficial result in a patient that is due not just to the treatment, but to the patient's expectations *about* the treatment.[12]

Blinded, controlled studies are the most reliable way to avoid bias in human medical research. *Blinded* means that patients won't know which treatment they'll be getting. The participants are split into groups, with all of them receiving a regimen — for example, a medication. But whereas one group receives the treatment that's being tested, the other group receives a sugar pill, or sham treatment, called a *placebo*.

This protocol helps determine how well a drug works and how much the patients' thoughts and beliefs (that they are taking a real drug) affect the treatment outcome. Researchers have to gauge to what degree the real treatment works because the subjects *think* that it will. As it turns out, our thoughts influence the treatment a lot. Brain imaging studies show that the placebo effect is physical. It changes bioneurological pathways in the brain, causing release of the reward and pain-relieving neurotransmitters, dopamine and endorphins.[13] Because this response is so consistent, research studies commonly factor it into their baselines. A fascinating study that looked at migraine and the triptan Maxalt found that pain intensity decreased when the drug was expected, even when participants received placebo. When Maxalt was administered but placebo was expected, the actual drug was not as effective.[14]

Even the people who administer a treatment can bias the results if they know who gets the real treatment and who gets the placebo. For that reason, *double-blinded* studies, in which neither patients nor researchers know who is getting what, are considered to be the most reliable. However, in a stunning 2011 randomized, controlled trial of irritable bowel syndrome by Harvard Medical School Professor of Medicine Ted J. Kaptchuk and colleagues, both researchers and participants actually knew if they were getting the real therapy or the placebo.[15] Remarkably, the placebo still worked to treat subjects' IBS, even though everyone knew they were getting a sham treatment!

We humans are very hopeful and imaginative creatures; our minds and beliefs can make us feel sick, or well. It's amazing how powerful the mind is!

Mind of a Champion

If thinking about a good outcome results in improvement, then can't we just think it *without* undergoing the treatment? Consider the true story of champion platform diver Laura Wilkinson.

Wilkinson had been a ten-time U.S. National Champion in women's ten-meter platform diving. Unfortunately, she suffered a serious injury during training six months before qualification rounds, downgrading her chances to make it to the 2000 Olympic Games in Sydney, Australia. She broke three bones in her foot and was unable to dive for two months during her recovery. A layoff this long can spell the end for athletes, who need to keep their muscles and form in top condition. Laura's sport required her to use her feet to push off from a three-story-high platform and flawlessly complete a dive. And it was her feet that were injured. Her chances didn't look good.

Cleverly, instead of physically practicing her dives during her recovery, Laura did the next best thing: she used mental imagery to practice her dives. In other words, she ran through them in her mind's eye and felt the action of diving in her body. Remarkably, she recovered in time to qualify for the Olympic team.

Maybe you watched the 2000 Olympics on television and remember watching her dive. China's team had won the event at seven of the last eight Olympics and was heavily favored to win the gold medal. No pressure there! But Laura Wilkinson won — the first American in thirty-six years to do so.

Laura's mental training helped her accomplish what she could not do physically when injured, and it propelled her to victory. Like a champion, you too can use your mental focus and the power of thought and belief to help your body relax and relieve your pain.

In Greek mythology, the warrior goddess Athena was most known for her wisdom and practical sense. Born wielding a sword, straight out of her father Zeus's headache, she had an independent spirit, was a fair and compassionate mediator, and tried to prevent war whenever possible. When necessary she fought bravely, assuming disguises and devising the Trojan Horse in opposition to a provocation to war. Athena never lost a battle.

I encourage you to be a warrior like Athena — a headache warrior — and pursue and attack your headaches, determined to win each battle and the larger war. If you lose your way, get right back on track and conquer your headaches with passion, creativity, and cunning. Be willing to do whatever it takes to be a warrior for your own health, and along the way, combat the inner and outer forces that seek to deter you from claiming your power to heal your headaches. It is the hero's journey.

Part Two

Handling
Headache Triggers

5 The Chinese Menu Theory

When I was forty-two years old, my migraines worsened, becoming so regular that I could predict my periods with them: each month I got a severe migraine the day before my period started. When I began learning stress reduction practices, that pattern changed, and most months my period would arrive without being announced by a disabling migraine.

I started comparing my heavy migraine months with those that were migraine-free and found that when I ate and slept better, drank more water, and was less stressed during the previous month, I would not get the migraine. The opposite was true when my previous month's activities were not as healthy. Perhaps you have noticed a similar pattern in how several things seem to add up to create your pain.

This led me to concoct the Chinese Menu Theory. The name goes back to my childhood in Los Angeles. On some Sunday nights, my family would go out to dinner at our favorite Chinese restaurant. We would order our food "family style," meaning each person would choose a dish from column A, a dish from column B, one from column C, and so on. All the delicious dishes of food would be brought out and placed on a lazy Susan in the middle of the table, and we would all partake of each dish to make up our meal.

In that same way, combinations of factors often add up to headaches, whereas one alone might not. Imagine that instead of ordering a family-style dinner, you are ordering your migraine from a menu of triggers. You could choose a potential trigger from column A — skipping meals, for example — which by itself may or may not produce your migraine. You could choose one from column B — for instance, lack of sleep — and again, you might get a migraine, maybe not. Choose another from column C — perhaps shoulder tension — and you may or may not get a migraine. From column D, we'll choose stress; perhaps you will get that migraine, perhaps you won't. But...if you combine items from columns A and B; B and C; A and D; A, B, C, *and* D, and so on...together they would add up to create your personal migraine stew.

Sample Migraine Triggers Menu

COLUMN A	COLUMN B	COLUMN C	COLUMN D
Skipping meals	Lack of sleep	Shoulder tension	Stress

My most reliable trigger combo used to be hours of chewing gum while clothes shopping, plus no water or lunch. (Who needs food?) My energy was powered by dopamine, the feel-good hormone that shopping produced in my brain. It was fun while it lasted, but my jaw was working overtime, combined with everything else, and the next day's migraine would make me regret it.

Everything Counts

This program works because we consider everything that might trigger a headache — and in all domains.

If you have tried a number of individual self-care strategies with limited success, including a variety of natural methods, it could be that you're not looking at everything. For example, you might have quit caffeine or eliminated entire categories of foods, such as wheat or dairy products. Then your headaches continued, so you ruled those items out as triggers and put them back into your diet. After all, eliminating them seemingly had no effect. Or perhaps you tried massage or meditation to reduce your stress but concluded they weren't helpful because your headaches persisted.

That's where the Chinese Menu Theory comes in: it addresses your whole self. You are not just what you eat or drink or your exercise routine or your stress. You are all of it combined. By taking everything in your life together as a whole — diet, lifestyle, posture, thinking, mood, stressors, and so on — you can gain new insights into how your triggers add up to your headaches.

Common Headache Triggers

The following list of headache triggers is adapted and expanded from one first published in *Migraine: The Complete Guide* by the American Council on Headache Education (Dell, 1994).[1] It's usefully arranged by category — dietary, environmental, lifestyle, physical, medication, and hormonal — so you can mine each area for clues and look at your life as a whole. You might notice this list is similar to but more extensive than the one you completed in the personal profile in chapter 3.

Lists of headache triggers are subjective. You are a unique individual, a delicate balance of chemistry with a history and an emotional life. What affects you might not affect me and vice versa. With some triggers, quantity also counts: a small amount of chocolate, wine, or exercise might not trigger your migraine, but a larger serving or a longer workout just might.

Perhaps you will recognize some of your triggers and rule out others from the list. Perhaps you aren't certain, or have no idea. For now, simply read it and see if anything rings a bell.

Headache Triggers

Dietary
additives,
  preservatives
aged cheese
alcoholic beverages
artificial sweetener
avocado
banana
beans
beer
caffeine
chocolate
citrus fruit
corn
dairy products
fermented food
food allergy
food sensitivity
garlic
high-fructose corn
  syrup
honey
hot dogs
lack of caffeine
lack of water
liquor
low blood sugar

luncheon meat
MSG
nuts
onion
pickled food
skipping meals
sour cream
sourdough bread
soy sauce
spicy food
sugar
wheat gluten
wine
yogurt

Environmental
air pollution
bright light
chemical sensitivity
dim light
dry air
excessive cold
excessive heat
flashing light
fluorescent light
fumes
high altitude

high humidity
hot, dry wind
loud noise
low barometric
  pressure
mold, mildew
motion
optical pattern
perfume
scents
secondhand smoke
stormy weather
strong odor
too much sun
weather changes

Lifestyle
anxiety
cigarette smoking
commuting
disrupted sleep
excessive sleep
fatigue
insufficient food
insufficient sleep
irregular eating
let-down headache

recreational drug use
routine change
stress
traveling

Physical
cold, flu, virus
exercise
exertion from sex or
   sports
head trauma
lack of exercise
medical procedure
posture and
   ergonomics
sinusitis, rhinitis
temporomandibular
   joint dysfunction
   (jaw tension and/or
   pain)

tension, tightness,
   pain (in shoulders,
   neck, head, face)
unsupportive bed,
   pillow
vision problems
   (eyestrain)

Medication
analgesic, simple
   (overuse)
analgesic, combina-
   tion (overuse)
anti-asthma medicine
anticonvulsant
antidepressant
blood pressure
   medicine
blood vessel dilator
diuretic

drug "cocktail"
   (combining several
   medications)
ergotamine (overuse)
opioid (overuse)
triptan (overuse)

Hormonal
birth
birth control (pills,
   patch, IUD)
hormone replacement
   therapy
menarche
menopause
menstrual cycle
ovulation
perimenopause
postpartum
pregnancy

Bodies Change over Time

In trying to solve your headache mystery, also consider that bodies change over time. The factors that cause your headaches now
might not be the same as those that triggered them originally. For
example, some habits that we had as teenagers or young adults are
unsustainable as we get older, at least not without consequences.

Perhaps your headaches began in college, when you would
stay up all night studying and writing papers while unconsciously
torquing the position of your head, neck, and back. Your younger,
more pliable body might have suffered yet bounced back easily. But
with age, bodies become less resilient, and recovery time lengthens.
Irregular eating habits or food choices, which did not take a toll in

your youth, could still influence your choices today. But whereas a skipped meal or snack back then just made you feel weak, dizzy, or grouchy, the same behavior now results in a bad migraine.

Just One More Thing

Keep the ideas in this chapter in mind as you read chapters 6 through 10, where you'll learn more about specific triggers and how to track them. In these chapters, you'll notice that some triggers receive more attention than others and that they're listed in order of the most commonly troublesome rather than in alphabetical order. Although each person's triggers and combinations of factors are different, certain triggers appear to be universally problematic — yet headache sufferers might give them less exploration than needed. You might be surprised to find that your triggers are different than what you thought they were.

6 Dietary Triggers

What you eat (or don't eat) matters, especially when it comes to migraine. Migraine sufferers can be sensitive to alcohol, caffeine, sugar, skipping meals, lack of water, MSG, preservatives, artificial dyes, flavorings, sweeteners, hot dogs, cured meats, aged and fermented foods, dairy products, wheat gluten, spicy foods, and amines. This chapter delves into these triggers and more.

The purpose of identifying and tracking your food triggers is to uncover your personal migraine cause and effect. Some of the foods discussed in this chapter will likely affect you, and others will not. If you are not sensitive to a food that you enjoy, such as wheat or dairy, despite its presence on a migraine triggers list, then keep it in your diet. For example, cottage cheese and Greek yogurt are widely available sources of high-quality protein that are easy to grab on the run. Don't eliminate a (healthy) food you enjoy just because it is on a list. Track your diet and find out.

Foods and drinks can trigger migraines for a variety of reasons. If you drink a glass of wine and get a migraine, your trigger could be the alcohol, the sulfites, the naturally occurring tyramine, or a combination of these...or perhaps you didn't eat enough protein that day. There can be additional variables in the equation that determine how, why, when, and where a particular trigger will affect you. For example, quantity can matter. Two glasses of wine or three squares of dark chocolate might be too much, whereas one might be fine. That is why tracking your food and drink intake is so important, and why elimination diets (in which you eliminate most foods and then add them back one by one to identify which are your triggers) are usually unnecessary.

Working with diet is an extremely important part of managing migraine in particular, and chapter 9, "Diet for Migraine Prevention," discusses this topic in detail, with a complete plan for how to work with foods and meal times. And eating healthfully is good for everyone, even people with headache types not triggered by diet.

Alcohol

Red wine, beer, and liquor are potent migraine triggers, and drinking alcoholic beverages can be hit or miss, even in small amounts. The culprit can be alcohol itself, or the sugars, coloring agents, by-products of fermentation called *congeners*, tannins in grape skins, sulfites, or tyramine. Individuals vary in the kinds, brands, grades, and vintages they can tolerate. Eating protein and drinking water throughout the day before taking those sips with dinner can sometimes help. Some people with tension-type headache say that drinking an occasional beer, glass of wine, or cocktail eases their tension and helps them relax.

If you are willing to suffer the consequences, you can experiment with clear-colored spirits like tequila or vodka, organic white wine, or prosecco. You just have to decide if it's worth the risk.

Sherri's story shows how unpredictable alcohol can be for those who are sensitive to it. She and her husband enjoyed pairing California wines with food until she realized they were connected to her chronic migraines. After three months of sessions with me, Sherri was migraine-free. She was eating well, drinking lots of water and no wine, and didn't need her relief drug, sumatriptan. One evening at a restaurant, she and her husband took a chance and shared a bottle of white with dinner. Ecstatic that she didn't get a migraine and thinking she was safe, they ordered a case from the vineyard the following day.

Guess what happened? When the wine they ordered arrived and Sherri had a glass, she got a horrible migraine.

What went wrong? She had eaten well that day and paired the wine with food, just like at the restaurant. Could the problem have been grapes from a particular vineyard, perhaps one of many that contributed to that batch or vintage? Were there different growing conditions, barrels, fertilizers, herbicides, or fungicides that could have affected the wine? We will never know, but Sherri's story illustrates the delicate balance of factors that headache triggers can be.

Even the alcohol contained in foods can be a trigger. I got a memorable migraine from a widely distributed brand of soy sauce that is commonly available at health food stores. I thought it would be safe because the store did not carry products with MSG or preservatives. When I later checked the label, I noticed it contained alcohol. It couldn't have been much, but it was enough for me. I now use only naturally brewed soy sauce that does not contain alcohol.

I learned that one brand of a product might trigger a migraine, but another might not. I could have concluded that soy sauce was the problem and eliminated it completely. Instead, by examining the label, I realized it was the alcohol and was able to find a brand without it that didn't trigger my migraine — when used in moderation.

Caffeine, Caffeine Withdrawal, and Chocolate

Did you know that caffeine is regulated as a drug? Caffeine and caffeine withdrawal are among the most potent and underrated triggers. Caffeine-containing beverages and foods include coffee, espresso, tea (black, orange pekoe, green, white), colas, soft drinks, energy drinks, and chocolate. Even decaf contains a small amount. Many over-the-counter (OTC) pain preparations, such as Excedrin and Anacin, and prescription headache drugs, like Cafergot and Fiorinal, contain caffeine.

People are often unaware of the amount of caffeine hidden in the everyday foods they consume. A two-ounce square of dark chocolate contains about forty grams of caffeine, the equivalent of a shot of espresso. Let's not forget chocolate in beverages, ice cream, frozen yogurt, toppings, cookies, cakes, and brownies.

Table 1 provides generic measures of the caffeine contained in some foods, drinks, and medicines. Note that caffeine content will vary with brands and brew times.[1] A simple internet search will yield more specific content information for most brands on the market.

Have you ever heard the advice that drinking a cup of strong coffee can ward off a migraine? According to one theory of migraine pain, the reason this works is that blood vessels in your head and face dilate as a result of neurochemical reactions in your brainstem. The inflamed vessels then disturb the nerves around them. Caffeine constricts those blood vessels and reverses the inflammation.

The problem is that regular consumption of one or more cups per day can cause a rebound effect, when that intake is skipped or delayed and the constricting caffeine wears off, which can happen within twenty-four hours.

How much caffeine do you consume daily? If you are a regular coffee or tea drinker and wake up with headaches each morning (or get them on weekends when you sleep later), caffeine could be the problem. Regular intake above the level your body can handle is one way that an episodic migraine can become chronic. The following anecdotes from my client files show how insidious caffeine can be.

In her Headache Diary (see chapter 10), my client Barbara

Table 1. Caffeine Content in Foods and Medicine

Product	Amount	Caffeine (mg)
Coffee, brewed	8 ounces	80–135
Coffee, drip	8 ounces	115–175
Coffee, decaffeinated	8 ounces	3–4
Espresso	1 shot	50
Espresso, decaffeinated	1 shot	4
Black tea, brewed	8 ounces	40–60
Green tea, brewed	8 ounces	15
White tea, brewed	8 ounces	15
Iced tea, bottled	12 ounces	9–32
Soft drinks and colas, caffeinated	12 ounces	34–56
Energy drinks (e.g., Red Bull)	8.2 ounces	80
Hot cocoa	8 ounces	14
Dark chocolate	1 ounce	20
Anacin, maximum strength	2 tablets	64
Excedrin, Excedrin Migraine	2 tablets	130
Midol Menstrual Complete	2 caplets	120
Fiorinal, Fioricet	2 tablets	80
Cafergot	2 tablets	200

reported drinking two cups of black tea per day, which seemed fine upon first glance. But when she wasn't migraine-free after implementing most of the Mundo Program, we started mining more deeply for clues. Only then did she sheepishly admit that she used three tea bags to brew each cup. We already knew that she took two Excedrin almost daily, in total making her caffeine intake the equivalent of five to six cups of coffee per day. No wonder Barbara would wake up in the morning with full-blown migraines! Her honest revelation was the breakthrough that she needed in order to progress.

Lily, a hairstylist and stay-at-home mom, was referred by her neurologist to my six-week medical center class for her daily migraines. Every day for fourteen years, Lily had taken two extra-strength Excedrin tablets containing 130 milligrams of caffeine, the equivalent of a strong cup of coffee. I suggested that she was getting a rebound effect as the caffeine in the Excedrin wore off each morning. Although she was in pain every day, Lily was sure that the medication was the only thing keeping her from more pain. She feared, and rightly so, that if she stopped taking it, her headaches would get worse. I suggested that she stair-step down super slowly, but her fear kept her stuck, and she continued her daily dosage throughout the remainder of the class. In light of that, I was delighted to receive a note from her two months later:

> Dear Jan,
>
> Since your seminar, little by little, I've been getting off Excedrin and am now in my third week without it. I feel like my headache cycle is broken. It's exciting! Not only that, but the irritable bowel syndrome that had bothered me for so long is gone.
>
> Thank you,
> Lily

We live in a fast-paced world, and an enjoyable social culture has mushroomed up around coffee and tea drinking. Caffeine boosts energy and mood levels, so if you enjoy a little caffeine, I fully understand. However, you have to find the right amount for your body, which is the amount you can have without getting a migraine when you skip it. And watch out for caffeine creep: a morning two-shot espresso drink could be your limit, but when an afternoon pick-me-up espresso, cup of tea, or iced tea with lunch becomes a habit, giving you a migraine if you skip or delay it, you are over your limit.

Sugar, Skipping Meals, and Low Blood Sugar

Sugars, including white and brown sugar, high-fructose corn syrup, corn syrup, cane sugar, honey, agave syrup, stevia, molasses, sorghum, coconut palm sugar, and maple syrup, can trigger migraine because they affect blood sugar levels, as does skipping meals. Because this topic is crucial in migraine management, we will cover it in depth in chapter 9.

Lack of Water

Water drinking helps prevent headaches, and lack of water is a common trigger. People don't drink enough water for a variety of reasons. Many people are unaware of their thirst, simply ignore it, or do not prepare for situations in which drinking water is not readily available. For example, a quick errand can turn into a few hours without water, or you don't drink water for hours before bedtime because you don't want to have to get up in the middle of the night to go to the bathroom.

Your body loses water in all climates. During the summer you sweat it out due to heat, and in winter it evaporates due to cold temperatures outdoors and heating indoors. In gyms, we work out year-round and sweat while we're doing it, and caffeinated and alcoholic beverages are also dehydrating. To keep your system lubricated and humming and your digestion and elimination working smoothly, you should drink a minimum of two quarts of water per day, which is sixty-four ounces. A two-liter water bottle holds almost sixty-eight ounces. In winter, it helps to humidify the air — you can do this by placing a glass or stainless-steel bowl of water on or near your radiator or heat source. When the water is nearly evaporated, clean the bowl thoroughly with a scrubby and soap, then refill with water and return it to its location.

MSG, Food Additives, Preservatives, and Artificial Sweeteners

The chemical additives used in many foods and drinks can produce an instant migraine in many migraineurs.

Monosodium glutamate (MSG) is a flavor enhancer, sometimes identified on ingredient lists as "natural seasoning." It is commonly used in canned soups, soy sauce, Chinese food, and packaged or powdered salad dressings, gravies, and sauces. "No MSG" at a Chinese restaurant can still mean you have to request that the kitchen leave it out — and some ingredients might still contain it, unbeknownst to the staff.

MSG is a potent trigger for me, and even with precautions, I've awoken on many mornings the day after Chinese food with a blazing migraine, attributable only to MSG. It's like injecting a migraine directly into my bloodstream. And it doesn't matter if the food was cheap, expensive, or vegetarian. I used to give a restaurant two chances, but no more. My body doesn't lie. If I get a migraine, I don't go back. Life is too short to suffer from the avoidable.

Many packaged foods contain chemical preservatives, flavorings, colorings, or additives to which you could be sensitive. If you get a migraine after eating prepared foods you used to safely enjoy, such as fig bars, marshmallows, microwave popcorn, packaged snacks, or ginger ale, read the label — the manufacturer might have added a new chemical ingredient that you are sensitive to. So many fun foods have red, green, blue, and yellow food coloring in them. Just say no. Same with artificial sweeteners; research shows that artificial sweeteners in drinks, foods, dietary supplements, candies, and gum actually do not make us thinner — and they're chemicals!

Hot Dogs and Cured Meats

Foods that contain sodium nitrite or nitrate are triggers for many migraineurs. Sodium nitrite is a preservative that gives hot dogs, bacon, bologna, corned beef, and other smoked and cured meats their characteristic pink color.

If you enjoy these foods but they trigger your migraines, carefully check labels and eat only those meats that are naturally smoked, uncured, or cured without nitrites. Find the brands that work for you. Some people choose to stay away from these foods altogether, or go with "fake meats" made from tofu, wheat protein, grains, nuts, and veggies.

Aged and Fermented Foods

Aged cheeses, soy sauce, and fermented and pickled foods are similar in that they are either aged or inoculated with a culture. Other foods in this category include sourdough bread, aged or cured meats, tap beer, pickles, kimchi, sauerkraut, Marmite, and baking and brewer's yeast. For people who are sensitive to fermented products, even naturally brewed soy sauce can be problematic.

One reason these foods trigger migraine is that they contain high levels of a natural protein called *tyramine*. Tyramine is created from the breakdown of tyrosine, an amino acid that regulates neurotransmitters and adrenal, pituitary, and thyroid hormones. Tyramine is broken down in the stomach by monoamine oxidase (MAO), and headache patients who take a class of antidepressants called *MAO inhibitors* should avoid foods and supplements that contain tyramine.[2]

Dairy Products

Dairy is a mixed bag for chronic migraine sufferers, and everyone handles it differently. Some people are not sensitive to it. For those who are, it can cause bloating, gas, upset stomach, or excessive mucus — and it might or might not trigger their migraines.

Dairy triggers include aged and non-aged products, such as cow and goat milk, hard and soft cheeses, cottage cheese, goat cheese, sour cream, yogurt, and ice cream.

If you like dairy but are not sure how your body handles it, you can track it in your Headache Diary (see chapter 10). Perhaps you can't tolerate cow *milk* but are okay with yogurt. If you like dairy and it isn't a trigger for you, then leave it in your diet and adjust the type and portions to suit your digestion.

Gluten

Gluten is the protein of the grain and gives dough its stretchy, cohesive quality. Wheat (including spelt, kamut, farro, and durum) is the main ingredient in most pastas, breads, muffins, cakes, pastries, cookies, crackers, and flour tortillas. As with dairy, some people notice that gluten is a trigger — or find they are sensitive to it and feel better without it, migraine trigger or not. Barley, rye, and triticale also contain gluten, whereas corn, millet, rice, sorghum, amaranth, buckwheat, quinoa, and (technically) oats do not. You might be sensitive to one type of gluten and not another.

Some migraine patients eliminate gluten, as they do dairy, simply because it's on a list of triggers. If you enjoy and can easily digest wheat or other gluten-containing products without triggering a migraine, don't worry about giving them up. As part of a balanced diet, whole grains are beneficial because they help stabilize blood sugar levels and provide important nutrients.

You may have heard of celiac disease, and if gluten triggers your migraines you might wonder if you have it. Don't worry. Celiac disease and true gluten allergy are not the same as a gluten sensitivity that triggers migraine or IBS. An allergist or a nutritionist can test you for celiac disease, a genetic, potentially life-threatening autoimmune disorder that renders wheat indigestible. If gluten triggers your migraines, chances are you do not have celiac. (See "Food Allergy and Food Sensitivity" below.)

Whether gluten triggers your migraines, you are sensitive to it, or you must stay away from it because you have celiac or an allergy, the good news is that gluten-free breads, pastas, and a variety of baked goods made from rice, corn, chickpea (garbanzo bean), buckwheat, and amaranth flours have become more commonly available in grocery and health food stores and online. Or you can make your own goods at home from scratch or a mix.

Spicy Foods

Spicy foods, such as garlic, onions, and hot peppers, are less common headache triggers, but they give some people indigestion. If your indigestion keeps you awake at night and disrupts your sleep cycle, contributing to your migraine, try skipping spicy and highly seasoned foods, or use them in moderation.

Amines

Who knew an orange could trigger a migraine? Citrus fruits, nuts, beans, corn, bananas, avocados, yogurt, and sour cream all contain amines, which are part of the tyramine family. Amine content increases as these foods ripen and age.

Although these foods are less troublesome than others for most migraineurs, it could be that one of these amine-rich foods is triggering your migraines. Another may not. If you are not sensitive to foods containing amines, don't eliminate them from your diet — they provide good nutritional value in the form of protein, fiber, and healthy fats. Again, there's a difference between a sensitivity and an allergy. Some people are allergic to nuts, like peanuts or walnuts, and allergy is a different reaction than triggering a migraine (see next section).

Food Allergy and Food Sensitivity

Food allergies are not known to trigger migraine, and allergy is different than food sensitivity or intolerance. A food allergy causes a severe and immediate reaction in your immune system and can be life threatening. Even eating a small amount of the offending food can give an allergic person intense stomach cramps and diarrhea, and can cause the lips, face, neck, and/or throat to swell dangerously.

On the other hand, some people are *sensitive* to certain foods, brands, or varieties, which could then contribute to triggering their migraines. Keeping a Headache Diary can help you to discover if you have food sensitivities.

7   Environmental, Lifestyle, and Physical Triggers

*D*o environmental, lifestyle, and physical triggers contribute to your headaches? You might be surprised at how many of these triggers permeate your daily life. This chapter tackles specific triggers in these categories and gives solutions for managing them even when they seem to be outside your control.

Triggers that can lurk in your environment, in what you see, smell, and hear, include bright sunlight and fluorescent lighting; perfume, scents, and odors; and extremely loud noise or music. Weather changes, high altitude, and low barometric pressure are also commonly noted triggers.

Lifestyle matters. Day-to-day stress, insufficient sleep, irregular eating, secondhand smoke, smoking, stressful commutes, changes in your routine, and travel can all take their toll.

Physical triggers are large contributors to tension, migraine, and combination headaches, and this chapter explains in detail how and why this occurs. These triggers include upper body tightness, face and jaw tension, temporomandibular joint dysfunction (TMJ/TMD), poor posture and ergonomics, exercise and lack of it, exertion, sex, unsupportive bed and pillow, sinusitis, vision problems, cold, flu, virus, head trauma, and medical procedures.

Remember to consider the triggers in this chapter when you

begin keeping your Headache Diary in chapter 10. Then, in addition to the solutions mentioned in this chapter, you can find more answers in part 3 of this book, which teaches meditation, breathing, gentle exercises, and other practices to address stress-related, postural, and physical triggers. Part 4 gives detailed self-massage instructions for easing your tension, pain, and headaches.

Environment

Although it might seem you have little control over your environment, with awareness and preparation you can take practical steps to protect yourself. For example, if you are sensitive to heat, sun, and bright light, you can make a habit of wearing or carrying sunglasses and a hat with a brim, and bringing along a water bottle.

Visual Triggers

Sun, glare, bright light, dim light, fluorescent lighting, flashing lights, optical patterns and effects, GIFs, and certain video games can trigger migraine.

It's worth noting that the fluorescent lighting often used in institutional and industrial buildings has a flicker rate of 60 cycles per second (CPS), which bothers some migraine sufferers. The higher flicker rate of compact fluorescent lamps (CFL) is reportedly less likely to be a trigger, but research is needed. There's speculation that light-emitting diodes (LEDs) might even be worse because their flickering light dims 100 percent rather than the lower 35 percent dimming of CFLs.[1]

Solutions

Protect yourself from bright or flickering lights and intense optical effects. Shade your eyes from bright sun and glaring snow with sunglasses and a hat. Use sun visors in the car, walk in the shade, and block or filter direct sunlight. Avoid squinting. Change interior lighting, improve where you sit relative to the light — rearrange or move your office if need be. Give your eyes some exposure to sunlight when you don't have a migraine, so you don't become overly sensitive to it by always blocking it.

Temperature

Is it too hot, too cold, or just right for you? Your body loses moisture in both hot and cold indoor and outdoor climates. But cold can be a particularly powerful trigger; when your body is cold, your muscles and fascia contract in protection, producing upper body tension that leads to migraine and tension headaches. Don't forgo a sweater, jacket, scarf, or long pants in winter just because you think you're hardy, and don't ignore chilly summers in places like San Francisco or disregard air-conditioning that blows cold air on your neck and shoulders.

SOLUTIONS

Stay hydrated in all temperatures. When it's hot, stay out of the sun and keep exposure to a minimum. Walk in the shade, use an umbrella at the beach and air-conditioning at home and in your car, avoid outdoor peak temperature times, and wear breathable, natural-fiber clothing.

Gear up for the cold! Always wear a hat, scarf, and gloves along with your coat or jacket to keep your head, neck, upper back, shoulders, and hands warm and cozy — especially when it's damp or windy. That goes for indoors too, and if you feel chilled, wear socks and slippers. Layer your clothing. Keep a bowl of water on or near the heat source to humidify the air.

Control for indoor temperature extremes. Turn air-conditioning down or off, move to a less chilly or drafty location in the room or switch rooms, and wear a sweater and scarf — even in summer if needed.

Scents, Odors, and Chemical and Environmental Sensitivity

Does your job, your hobby, or a trip to the nail salon expose you to fumes, scents, or chemicals? Scented products, both artificial and natural, are so pervasive that they are easy to ignore, but strong odors, perfumes, and other scents can make migraineurs like me swoon. Repeated exposure to one or multiple chemicals over time can make you develop chemical sensitivities. In some cases, a lack of exposure can also create sensitivity; I became sensitive to perfumes and scents after many years of attending fragrance-free events.

Consider the personal products used daily by you and by people around you, such as soap, lotion, shampoo, conditioner, hair-styling products, makeup, perfume, cologne, deodorant, nail polish, polish remover, and hand sanitizer. Everyday household and car products emit scents, odors, and fumes. Pay attention to dish and laundry soap, fabric softener, dryer sheets, disinfectant, cleaners, fabric shampoo, bleach, furniture polish, air freshener, candles, and incense.

Does the smell of paint, paint remover, thinner, sealant, or wax bother you? Do you gag, like me, from fumes at the gas station? Petroleum and resin-based products can be potent triggers. After decades of migraines, my artist client gave up her oil-based paints and thinners for water-based acrylics and suffered no more.

We live in a veritable chemical stew. That "fresh car smell" when you buy a new car, not to mention the smells of a new sofa, mattress, pillow, or carpet, is the result of outgassing, meaning the odors produced by the chemicals emitted by foam, latex, plastic, resin, and glue. Lawn, garden, and farming products, including fertilizer, herbicide, insecticide, and chemical solvent, are not only toxic — they also give off strong odors and fumes. Environmental mold and mildew and secondhand cigarette smoke are also in this category.

Even nature herself, in the form of dust, pollens, and grasses, can cause an inflammatory response that then contributes to your Chinese menu of headache triggers.

SOLUTIONS

Use natural, unscented personal and household products when possible. Note that even unscented products (for instance, unscented fabric softener dryer sheets) trigger some people's migraines. Wear a mask or use a ventilator when working with petroleum and resin-based products. Do at-home manicure-pedicures. Work in well-ventilated areas or outdoors. Seek out products and brands that don't bother you; stay away from dust, pollens, and grasses; and limit your exposure.

On the positive side, your nose and body are warning you that something in your environment is irritating your system. Avoid, eliminate, clean up, and treat the source of cigarette smoke, chemical, and mold-based triggers, which can also cause other health issues.

Loud Noise

Loud noise, like noise from city streets, construction, or a rock concert, triggers migraine for some people.

SOLUTIONS

Wear earplugs or noise-canceling headphones to dampen the sound, situate yourself away from loudspeakers, close windows, use a white noise machine, and avoid loud environments if they bother you.

Weather, Altitude, and Motion

Many migraineurs report a strong connection between their headaches and the weather, including low barometric pressure, changes in pressure and temperature before a storm, high humidity, dry air in winter, and hot desert winds, as well as smog and air pollution. Other triggers include high altitude and motion in cars, planes, and boats.

It may be that regions with more stable weather patterns, with fewer variations, are better for people with migraine. This can be difficult to measure, however, since how the weather affects you is an individual thing and depends on the other factors contributing to your migraines.

SOLUTIONS

Although you can't change the weather, it is less likely to affect you when all your other ducks are in a row, meaning your life is balanced and other triggers are handled. Be prepared by following forecasts, and chart and learn your weather triggers. The solutions in the "Temperature" section above also apply here. Some migraineurs go to the extreme of moving to a personally less-triggering climate.

When traveling to high-altitude areas, remedy potential headaches by eating leafy greens and taking supplements, like blue-green algae and kelp drinks or tablets, at least one week prior to your trip. If you suffer from motion sickness, avoid reading in the car, and look outside of the vehicle you're riding in.

Lifestyle

How does your daily lifestyle contribute to your headaches? Everyday activities that you take for granted can be a minefield of triggers.

Stress

You could say that a headache is nature's readout of all the stressors taxing your system. And who doesn't have stress at one time or another? Furthermore, even if you know you're stressed, you don't always know where it's held in your body or what to do about it. Admitting the problem and pinpointing it are the first steps to working with it.

For "thinkers" and "worriers," the energy of all that stress and anxiety goes straight to our shoulders, neck, head, and face and is held there as tension, tightness, and pain. In the Always versus Never exercise in chapter 4, your body reacted to your positive and negative thoughts as if they were real life. Whether your stress results from apprehension about things that *have* happened, *are* happening, or *might* happen, whether your stress is physical, mental, or emotional — if you ignore it, you will store it!

SOLUTIONS
Regular practices that build mind-body awareness, like breathing, meditation, and self-massage, described in parts 3 and 4, will help you stay centered under pressure and reduce upper body tension that contributes to headaches.

Sleep Problems

Not enough sleep, disrupted sleep, and irregular sleep-wake patterns often factor into migraine. To recover and recharge, your body needs sufficient sleep daily, usually eight hours, including high-quality REM sleep. Women in perimenopause and menopause can be particularly affected by sleep problems.

SOLUTIONS
Forgo afternoon caffeine! Exercise, but not too late in the day. Practice meditation, centered breathing, and whatever else helps you relax. Give yourself winding-down time before bed. (Be aware that alcoholic drinks can also disrupt sleep.) Take a warm bath and sip chamomile tea. Try a guided meditation, relaxation, or sleep recording.

Equip yourself with earplugs, sound-canceling earphones, or a white-noise machine. To block light, use an eye mask or heavy curtains, and turn off, turn around, turn over, or dim electronic devices and readouts. Go to sleep at a regular time, and aim to get seven to nine hours of uninterrupted quality sleep each night — and more for teenagers and children. Avoid sleeping later on weekends to "catch up" on your sleep because it disrupts your regular food and caffeine schedule.

Irregular Eating

As my grandma would say, "Did you eat?" Skipping breakfast or forgoing meals, having irregular and/or rushed mealtimes, and eating unhealthy foods can spell big trouble for migraine sufferers.

SOLUTIONS

In chapter 9, we will discuss the all-important connections between skipping meals, low blood sugar, diet, and migraine. Improving your dietary habits will transform your life!

Cigarette Smoking

Are you a smoker? Do you enjoy a cigarette with coffee? One speeds you up, while the other calms you down. From exposing you to the smoke fumes, chemicals, and nicotine to suppressing appetite and impairing breathing, cigarette smoking can contribute to migraine and other health conditions.

SOLUTIONS

Do whatever you can to stop smoking. Get assistance from your primary care provider, acupuncturist, hypnotherapist, or other professional.

Commuting

The ways in which you use your body to get to work, run errands, or otherwise get around can be part of your Chinese menu of triggers.

Whether you drive, bike, take public transportation, or walk, and whether you have a short or a long trip, commuting epitomizes how one activity can involve several triggers. Is this also true for other activities you do regularly?

Let's look at the multiple factors that go into commuting — posture, ergonomics, bright sun, stress, and dehydration — and examine some of their trouble spots.

DRIVING

- What is your driving posture? Leaning back to relax actually forces your neck and head forward so you can see the road, putting tension in your shoulders, upper back, neck, and arms. Straining forward to see over the steering wheel has the same effect on your upper body and forces your shoulders up. The tension created by postural misalignment builds into tightness, soreness, and pain and contributes to headaches.
- Does your stress skyrocket when you're driving? If you're stuck in traffic or getting a late start, do you unconsciously hold your breath, raise your shoulders, and grip the wheel? (I solved my sore shoulders mystery after catching myself actually pushing the steering wheel on road trips from L.A. to the Bay Area — as if to make the car go faster!)
- Do you squint and strain your eyes while driving during the day, at dusk, or at night?

BIKING, WALKING, AND MORE

- Biking, walking, and riding public transportation, which commuters often do in combination, can present many of the same problems as driving.
- When you're biking, your torso is often bent forward at the waist, forcing the back of your neck, skull, and shoulders to scrunch up so you can see the road.

- For any of these transportation modes, do you carry a heavy cross-body bag or backpack?

SOLUTIONS

- For driving and biking: Adjust your seat to fit your height and body type — and sit vertically. Consciously relax your arms and shoulders.
- For driving: Get a lumbar support and position it below your waist to support your lower back. Sit high enough to see over the steering wheel without craning your neck, tilting your chin up, or raising your arms and shoulders to hold the wheel.
- For all commutes: To improve your mood and reduce stress, plan ahead, get an earlier start, allow sufficient time, and listen to calming music. If possible, telecommute full- or part-time. Know your visual limits. Don't strain your forehead, eyes, and cheeks in response to dim light, dark, twilight, or extended driving time.

Routine Changes, Travel, and Let-Down

Travel and changes in your routine can take you out of your usual patterns of eating, drinking, and sleeping, which can also result in *let-down headache*.

When preparing for travel, school, a new job, or a major life event, most people get so busy that they don't sleep, eat, or hydrate as well as they normally would. Then when they're finally on vacation or the stressful event has passed and it's time to relax, that's when the migraine, called a *let-down headache*, strikes! Think of everything you go through to get to your destination: for example, traveling might include time zone changes, extended and uncomfortable plane, bus, or car seating, and carrying luggage.

SOLUTIONS

Reduce your load when you travel, hike, or backpack. Carrying heavy weight can cause tight neck and shoulders, leading to headaches. Travel with an inflatable neck pillow, pashmina-type scarf or shawl, and wheeled luggage and totes. In the midst of travel preparation and routine changes, try to stick to your healthy diet and sleep patterns.

Physical

Physical triggers are easy to identify once you start paying attention to them. They include upper body tightness and tension, poor posture, unsupportive bed and pillow, the way you carry your stuff, exercise or lack of it, and exertion. Cold, virus, flu, vision problems, head trauma, and medical procedures are also listed in this broad category.

In parts 3 and 4, you will learn mind-body practices and therapies to reduce tightness, tension, and pain and prevent it from building up. In part 5, we will explore how stress and tension in body and mind can stem from your emotional history.

Upper Body Tension, Tightness, and Pain

Shoulder, neck, head, and face tension, tightness, and pain are among the most common headache triggers. A single point or an entire area can feel tight and painful, causing you to immobilize it. When held in one position over time, by usage or unconscious habit, these tight points and surrounding areas become fixed, further restricting their movement. If you wonder why your shoulders or neck are always sore or why your tension headaches occur on certain days, look to your postural habits throughout your day, what you carry, and how you carry it.

SOLUTIONS

If you carry a heavy handbag, tote, computer case, briefcase, back-pack, or gym bag that has your "whole life in it," try lightening your load. Carry only what you really need in order to get from point A to point B, and assess what you carry daily. Lighten the load in your purse and wallet. Get a rolling briefcase, backpack on wheels, or shopping cart. Practice good posture, desk exercises, face play, and self-massage (see parts 3 and 4) to relieve and prevent tension, tightness, and pain.

Jaw Tension, TMJ/TMD

Jaw tension and soreness and "TMJ," the colloquial term for tem-poromandibular joint dysfunction (TMD), denotes pain in your jaw, the area directly in front of your ears. Jaw tension and TMJ affect people of all ages and can be an indication of teeth reposition-ing, bite misalignment, dental malocclusion, teeth grinding, and stress. Dental work, such as fillings, crowns, and extractions, can change your bite, chewing surfaces, and jaw positioning, which also affect your head and face muscles, fascia, ligaments, and tendons.

The joint between your upper jaw, or *maxilla*, and your lower jaw, or *mandible*, can become inflamed if you clench, grind, or gnash your teeth while asleep or awake or overexercise it by chewing gum. Teeth grinding during sleep, a condition called *bruxism*, is often an outlet for stress that can only be released when your conscious mind is at rest. Each clench or chew affects your jaw muscles, ligaments, tendons, and surrounding nerves, which also connect with other muscles that wrap around your head and temples.

SOLUTIONS

Try a plastic night guard to prevent teeth grinding, or consult with an orthodontist about getting braces or a retainer to adjust your bite. Breathing and meditation can also help with stress-related teeth grinding. In chapter 17, you can learn self-massage routines for relaxing your head and face.

Posture

Poor posture causes bodily tension and pain from misalignment and contributes to shallow breathing and decreased energy levels.

My headache clients present with a postural shape that is so consistent that I named it: the "C-curve." Viewed in profile, whether sitting or standing, the torso is shaped like the letter *C* — the result of holding the head and shoulders forward, collapsing the chest, and rounding the back.

We unconsciously use head-forward posture when leaning in toward the computer screen or car windshield or when wearing heavy backpacks. Emotional factors also contribute to how we carry ourselves; we might slump when feeling sad, depressed, or less confident. The weight of the head held out front makes upper body muscles and fascia work overtime.

Other troublesome postures include sitting with neck or body torqued sideways; using a desk chair or car seat that's too high, too low, or tilted back; and using desk chair armrests that are too high for your body.

Solutions

"Stack" your body, with ear, shoulder, and hip joint in vertical alignment. Pay attention to your vertical line during activities, and strengthen it with core-building exercises and centering practices. Improve your ergonomics: make your seating (desk, couch, car) and what you carry work for you and not vice versa. In chapter 13, you will learn how to combat the C-curve, and in chapters 15 and 16, you will learn self-massage to loosen the tightness that keeps you stuck.

Exercise, Exertion, Sports, and Sex

Yes, any vigorous, sustained exercise can relieve physical and emotional buildup that contributes to tension headaches. Exercise heats the body, circulates more energy, creates flexibility and fluidity, and causes the brain to release more endorphins (feel-good hormones) and less cortisol (stress hormones). Just don't try it during a migraine.

From a somatic viewpoint, a tightly held structure is like a contraction throughout the entire body, almost like a shell. The increased energy and muscle contraction created when exercising or exerting yourself vigorously push up against that tight structure and can't release, creating a boomerang effect that exacerbates the tightness. This unconscious overall tightness can contribute to your headaches.

SOLUTIONS

Exercise gently (see chapter 14) between migraine episodes, and do gentle self-massage to prevent muscle-tension buildup. Don't exercise vigorously to ward off a migraine. Explore sensual touch and tantric sex to release tension and build intimacy and communication.

Lack of Exercise

During a migraine attack, almost any activity becomes impossible. If you have been dealing with chronic migraine over time, you probably haven't felt like exercising for a while. If you've been inactive due to pain, your body might feel tight, weak, or low energy. This can create a vicious circle: the migraine keeps you from exercise, and the lack of exercise feeds into your migraine.

SOLUTIONS

Of course, the antidote is exercise. It promotes well-being by increasing blood and lymph circulation, metabolizing your food, releasing waste, and enhancing your mood and energy levels. It heats up your muscles and expends your physical energy, which is helpful if you have trouble sleeping. Chapter 14 covers gentle ways to exercise for prevention without activating a migraine.

Unsupportive Bed and Pillow

If you consistently wake up with headaches or neck and shoulder stiffness and pain, look to your bed or pillow. Sleeping on an unsupportive bed, pillow, or both — whether too soft or too hard — is an oft-unheralded trigger. Although this is posture-related, I have given it its own category because we spend one-third of our lives sleeping (not even counting resting and lying down).

SOLUTIONS
Chapter 13, "Posture, Ergonomics, and Sleep," covers correct sleeping and lying-down postures to place your body in a neutral position, and there you can also find tips for choosing supportive bedding.

Sinusitis/Rhinosinusitis and Rhinitis

Sinusitis, now often termed *rhinosinusitis*, and *rhinitis* are conditions involving inflammation of the paranasal sinuses, or cavities, adjacent to the nose, cheeks, and eyes. Symptoms of rhinosinusitis are sinus pain and tenderness, headache, swelling, congestion, and thick, discolored nasal discharge.

Sinusitis can be caused by viral or bacterial infection. Viral sinusitis, also known as the common cold, is the most prevalent type and will typically resolve in seven to ten days. Bacterial sinusitis, which can develop from a viral infection, might require antibiotics.

Rhinitis affects 60 million people in the United States. *Nonallergic rhinitis* is caused by polyps, deviated septum, environmental pollutants such as cigarette smoke, or decongestant overuse.

Allergic rhinitis is caused by allergies to pollens, molds, dust mites, animal hair, industrial chemicals, pollutants, tobacco smoke, foods, medicines, and insect venom. Seasonal rhinitis, or hay fever, affects people at certain times of year (when ragweed is flowering). With perennial allergic rhinitis, people are affected all year (for example, when exposed to dust mites). Symptoms of allergic rhinitis are sinus pressure, nose irritation, sneezing, itching, congestion, eye irritation — and so-called sinus headache.

Because migraine and allergic rhinitis headache can have similar symptoms, patients are often misdiagnosed (or misdiagnose themselves) with sinus headache when they actually have migraine. Some studies show that up to 90 percent of patients and their doctors have it wrong.[2]

People with allergic rhinitis who get accompanying headaches often turn to nasal sprays, drops, and decongestants to ease nasal drip or sinus pain and congestion. However, daily or frequent use can result in overly dry nasal passages and habituation if the spray contains the medication oxymetazoline. Migraine that is misdiagnosed as a sinus condition can also result in unnecessary surgical intervention.

Solutions

Natural home remedies for rhinitis and rhinosinusitis can be very effective. These include hot washcloth compresses, steamy showers, nose-breathing while bending over a bowl of steaming water with a towel over your head and the bowl, nasal irrigation with saline solution using a bulb syringe or neti pot, herbal formulations, and drinking plenty of fluids. Limit your exposure to dust, dust mites, and pollens, wear sunglasses outdoors, close windows, use air-conditioning, and don't use window fans that draw in outside air.

Vision and Sight

Uncorrected vision, using glasses or contacts with an outdated prescription, reading in dim light, straining to read fine print, or not wearing sunglasses in bright light can trigger headaches. All of these can cause you to habitually squint, frown, or furrow your brow, and the contraction around your eyes makes your face scrunch into a constantly held position.

SOLUTIONS

Correct for the vision problems listed. Read in sufficient light, and enlarge the font or use a magnifier. Use the self-massage routines for head and face in chapter 17, which will help relieve unconscious facial tension.

Cold, Flu, Virus

Migraines often accompany cold, flu, or virus with fever, but these are typically occasional unless you are dealing with a chronic illness.

SOLUTIONS

If you are surprised with a migraine after seeing steady improvement, do not panic or worry that you are backsliding. You could just be coming down with a cold, virus, or flu. Hydrate!

Head Trauma

Migraine is a common side effect of concussion and bodily trauma, and this side effect can persist after medical treatment has been completed and the brain and body have ostensibly recovered. The trauma of the accident, whether physical, mental, emotional, or spiritual, can assume a life of its own and live in the body until it's released or resolved.

SOLUTIONS

A whole-person approach can be beneficial, as shown by the following two examples:

John, a twenty-year-old who was attending a top university on a sports scholarship, was referred by the team neurologist because his migraines continued for six months after he suffered a concussion. They abated with diet, bodywork, and Mundo Method hands-on headache therapy. Meditation, breathing, and somatic coaching helped John feel calmer and overcome his feelings of family and personal pressure. Then he had an "aha" moment: he realized that when he ran, he was always "in his head," thinking and performing. So he shifted to "being in his body" and dramatically reduced his stress.

Kirstin, a thirty-year-old professional artist, was having a difficult time after sustaining a concussion from a serious bike accident in which she flew over the handlebars. The accident affected her on multiple levels long after her neurologist cleared her of the concussion; she had constant migraines and kept feeling and seeing in her mind's eye the experience of her accident. The traumatic memory was locked in her body, especially in her jaw. When she released her pent-up emotions of pain, anger, fear, frustration, blame, and helplessness about the accident through somatic bodywork and coaching, Kirstin's migraines ceased.

Medical Procedures

Like a concussion, a medical procedure and subsequent recovery can cause migraine. Triggers include the anesthesia; medications taken before, during, and after the procedure (or withdrawal from them); and the procedure itself, such as a spinal tap or spinal block.

Whether a medical procedure is planned or due to an emergency or an accident, you often have little control over the situation and your environment. You might be awash in feelings of anticipation, anxiety, and helplessness. As a migraine sufferer, you might be sensitive to triggers commonly found in medical settings, such as fluorescent lighting, strong odors, loudspeaker announcements, or the loud clicking noise during an MRI. If you're an inpatient, you might also suffer from interrupted sleep, post-surgery nausea and constipation from medication, and pre- or post-procedure fasting or limited diet.

SOLUTIONS

Do whatever you can to limit your stress. If you have a planned procedure, you can do these beforehand. Calm your body and mind by meditating. Create an affirmation that makes you feel good. You might say, "My procedure and recovery are going smoothly with minimal pain. I am blessed with vibrant health and well-being." Mitigate potential environmental triggers by wearing earplugs and a sleep mask. Request and receive the help you need from positive-minded, supportive family and friends.

Be aware of the side effects of pain medications when taken over time, as covered in chapter 8, and work with your doctor to limit your exposure. Use complementary nondrug pain control methods including acupuncture, Eastern and Western herbs and supplements, homeopathy, heat and cold therapies, energy work, Reiki, gentle bodywork, and meditation.

8 Medication and Hormonal Triggers

*L*ike all the triggers discussed in this book, medication and hormones are enormous and complicated topics. This chapter provides an introduction to them along with anecdotes from my case files to help you connect the dots.

In filling out your Headache History Questionnaire in chapter 3, you listed your headache medications as well as others, including birth control and hormone replacement. Be sure to track them in your diary — and note if and when you add, subtract, or change anything.

Medication Triggers

Taking medications for headaches on a regular basis can transform your occasional episodes into a chronic condition. These medications include analgesics, ergotamines, triptans, and off-label drugs, such as anticonvulsants and antidepressants.

Headache can also be a side effect of medications prescribed for other conditions, including blood vessel dilators, diuretics, nasal decongestants, antidepressants, allergy remedies, and asthma and blood pressure medications. When people take pain medications for an extended time due to an injury or after surgery, their current headaches can grow worse or they can develop headaches even if they did not previously have them.

In tracking your triggers, consider the medications you are taking and how they make you feel. Is there a correlation between them and your migraines — when you take them, when they wear off, or when you first started? Look up each medication online and read about the side effects. If headache or migraine is on the list, consider those medications in your Chinese menu of potential triggers.

Medication-Overuse Headache

Medication-overuse headache (MOH) results from taking acute and/or symptomatic treatment medication too often. It is classified as a *secondary* headache — that is, it is secondary to the primary headache for which the medication is being taken.

MOH was previously termed *transformed migraine, rebound headache, drug-induced headache,* and *medication-misuse headache.* The names may have changed, but the symptoms haven't: a dull, constant headache, day after day. The new term is somewhat controversial because *overuse* implies that patients are to blame for "getting hooked," when they are simply trying to relieve their pain or comply with medical advice.[1]

In a 2001 research study meta-analysis, neurologists Hans-Christoph Diener and Zaza Katsarava found that migraine medications used on ten or more days per month could cause rebound. This revelation was especially shocking because the new class of triptan drugs, then on the market for only ten years, was considered to be exempt from overuse, unlike its predecessors. The study found that even these medications, if used consistently over time, individually or in combination, lead to an increase in the frequency and intensity of the original migraine, lower the pain threshold, and render preventative drugs ineffective. Triptan-induced rebound is also different than ergotamine- or analgesic-overuse rebound be-cause, instead of a tension-type headache, it is described as a daily "severe and prolonged migraine attack."[2]

How Much Is Too Much?

How much use does it take to trigger MOH? Less than you might think. And the list of culprits is dizzying.

When people with headache or migraine regularly take acute treatment drugs on ten or more days per month for three months, they can get MOH. (That's only two and a half days per week.) With simple analgesics, MOH takes fifteen or more medication days per month for three months to develop.[3]

Following is an abbreviated list of medications that can cause MOH, according to the above parameters:

- Simple analgesics: acetaminophen (Tylenol), acetylsali-cylic acid (aspirin), nonsteroidal anti-inflammatory drugs (NSAIDs), ibuprofen (Advil, Motrin), and naproxen (Aleve)
- Combination analgesics: acetaminophen, aspirin, and caf-feine (Excedrin); aspirin, caffeine, and butalbital (Fiorinal); acetaminophen, caffeine, and butalbital (Fioricet, Esgic); and acetaminophen and butalbital (Phrenilin)
- Ergotamine (Cafergot, DHE): Side effects include nausea, gastrointestinal upset, and tingling and numbness in extrem-ities. Ergotamine should not be taken during pregnancy or if you are considering pregnancy.[4]
- Triptans: sumatriptan (Imitrex), zolmitriptan (Zomig), riza-triptan (Maxalt), eletriptan (Relpax), sumatriptan and naproxen sodium (Treximet), naratriptan (Amerge), frova-triptan succinate (Frova), and almotriptan malate (Axert)
- Opioids (short-acting analgesics derived from opium): co-deine with acetaminophen (Tylenol #3), hydrocodone with

acetaminophen (Vicodin), meperidine (Demerol), oxy-codone with acetaminophen (Percocet), hydromorphone (Dilaudid), and morphine. Side effects are physical and psychological dependence, where increased usage brings less effectiveness and requires increasing amounts to work.

When headache patients take several medications throughout the month, which many do, MOH can develop insidiously because medications have a synergistic effect in combination even if the dosage of each is below the level that would cause overuse. For example, by using different medications for relief (triptan, NSAID, analgesic, opioid), for prevention (antiepileptic), and for sleep (antidepressant), patients become susceptible. When regulated drugs like butalbital (a barbiturate) or an opioid are combined with caffeine and a simple analgesic in one pill, *combination-analgesic-overuse headache* can result. Prescribed for tension headache and migraine, these medications are especially problematic to withdraw from.[5]

Ironically, to combat MOH, patients must discontinue their medications following a carefully monitored regimen overseen by their prescribing physicians. Otherwise, they can experience withdrawal symptoms, including severe headache, gastrointestinal upset, irritable mood, restlessness, and insomnia. For intractable cases, in-patient headache centers offer a controlled setting to help patients withdraw from medications as a first step in treatment. MOH diagnosis is confirmed when the patient's headaches resolve or return to their premedication state within three months after discontinuing the medication(s) in question.

Do Your Research about Medications and Side Effects

Learn about what you are putting into your body. If you are reading this book, my guess is you want to travel the natural path, with the goal of eliminating headache medication.

Headache and migraine patients and their practitioners often go through a process of deduction to find the most effective medication or combination of medications. A doctor might prescribe one and then substitute it with another if it proves to be or becomes ineffective. It can take a while to find what works, and they all can have side effects.

Some drugs are prescribed *off-label*, meaning your doctor is prescribing them for a condition other than the ones they were designed to treat. Pay special attention to side effects for any off-label medicines you are taking. For example, the antiepileptic drug topiramate (Topamax) is often prescribed as a daily migraine preventative, but it comes with significant side effects: numbness and tingling in the extremities, nausea, diarrhea, fatigue, difficulty concentrating, anxiety, and memory, appetite, and weight loss. In some patients, it can produce decreased vision, suicidal thoughts, insomnia, and reduced sweating resulting in elevated body temperature.

Other common off-label preventatives are beta-blockers, tricyclic antidepressants, selective serotonin reuptake inhibitors (SSRIs), and serotonin norepinephrine reuptake inhibitors (SNRIs). In addition to the side effects that can occur when you're taking them, these drugs also have a host of serious withdrawal symptoms.

Here's a short list of side effects from extended use of over-the-counter (OTC) and prescription medications: damage to kidneys, liver, or gastrointestinal tract (acetaminophen, ibuprofen), nausea, vomiting, liver damage, tolerance (opioids), numbness, weakness, headache, nausea (ergotamine), and dizziness (triptans).

Be informed. Before you begin or stop taking any prescription or OTC drug, do some research to get the latest information regarding side effects. If headache is among them, and if it's a medication you take for another condition, work with your doctor to adjust the dosage or find a better remedy, for which headache is not a side effect.

Use the information from your research plus the advice of your doctor to determine your best course of action, especially when it comes to weaning off any medication. Ask questions during your appointments, get a second or third opinion if you are in doubt, and find a new practitioner if you are not satisfied. Many conditions can be alleviated by stress reduction strategies, hands-on therapies, healthy diet, and somatic practices instead of a pill.

How People Get Hooked Unwittingly

Vicky had managed her migraines for decades with a regimen of prescription drugs — one for relief, one for prevention, plus an OTC analgesic. She had also tried a variety of alternative therapies with mixed results. She sought my help for an alternative to medication therapy because she wasn't tolerating its side effects.

Vicky described an all-too-familiar cycle: She knew she wanted to lighten up on the medications, but she had what I call "fear of the next pain." She was afraid a full-blown migraine would strike if she stopped her regimen or put off taking her meds. Vicky was rightfully concerned, but the more she worried about the pain, the more her fear produced tension and holding throughout her entire body, making a migraine more likely. On her practitioner's advice to not wait and her own experience of what happened when she did wait, she had begun taking her rescue, or abortive, medication preemptively, and if that didn't work she would also take a couple of OTC pain relievers.

This fear-based reaching for medication wouldn't be so bad if Vicky's headaches abated, but they didn't. They continued for years. It's easy to get on that merry-go-round but hard to get off without having a substitute therapy to help you feel better. Patients can fall into a predicament that itself can be difficult to recognize and admit to: they follow instructions to take medication at first signs of a migraine, so that it doesn't escalate, but in this way their usage builds up, leading to MOH.

Medication Withdrawal

When medication is not helping and might even be perpetuating your headaches, it could be time to adopt a new strategy. At some point, people decide that the side effects are outweighing the benefits, or they see the connections between their migraines and their medications.

If you decide to stop using a prescription drug, it is essential to enlist your doctor's help with your goal. First, many medications require a gradual decrease over time to safely discontinue them, so take it slow. If you stop cold turkey or taper off too quickly, you could experience withdrawal symptoms (which also goes for caffeine), such as migraine, nausea, gastrointestinal upset, mood changes, and fatigue.

Second, if you want to cease medication for pain, make a clear statement of your intention. Your doctor might suggest replacing one medication with another, which is one way the cycle of relying on medication for pain gets perpetuated, along with your headaches. If you want to go in a more natural direction than your practitioner is willing to support, consider changing to one who will.

Motivated to conquer her migraines before her wedding, my client Karen had a difficult experience when she tried to withdraw from amitriptyline (Elavil), a tricyclic antidepressant often prescribed for migraine prevention. She had integrated self-care into her routine, her migraine episodes were reduced from daily to one per week, and, feeling enthusiastic about her improvement, she had decided to get off her medication. After consulting with her neurologist, who advised her it would be okay to stop all at once, she thought she was being judicious in taking a week to decrease from forty milligrams a day to zero. As a result, however, she had extreme withdrawal symptoms: a horrible migraine, lost appetite, insomnia, dizziness, and gastrointestinal upset.

Based on her doctor's advice, she thought she was tapering off slowly, so the symptoms scared her and made her think "This is my life without medication." She didn't realize she was having withdrawal. So she called her doctor and went back on the amitriptyline. If Karen had decreased her dosage more gradually, she likely would not have had such harsh withdrawal symptoms and as a result would not have resumed the medication when she was trying to do the opposite.

If this is your goal too, you must monitor how you feel during the process. Obviously, drugs have very powerful effects, and it is essential to pay close attention to *your* body and *your* symptoms, no matter what your doctor or a manufacturer advises. Although people have similarities, there is no one exactly like you, and each person reacts and responds in unique ways.

Practices, Not Prescriptions

It takes a strong commitment to make that mental connection between medication and migraine and extricate yourself from MOH. I've had clients who could clearly see in their diary entries and clearly feel in their bodies that their migraines arrived each night when the triptans wore off. However, even after getting down to one or two triptan days per week, their fears of being disabled would creep back. So they would take the triptan — and their usage and headaches would again increase.

A self-care program is similar to taking medication in that they both require you to do something. Just as a pill won't work if you don't take it, a self-care program won't work if you don't follow it. However, self-care is different than standard medical treatment, and even some alternative therapies, in that you are taking action yourself rather than relying on being fixed by someone or something else.

If you are used to taking medication for your pain, try a little experiment: Notice how you feel when you reach for your meds. What changes in your body, and where do you feel it? Clients often report having a sense of relief. Remember the placebo effect? That's basically what's happening here. You're fairly confident that relief is in sight, which immediately eases your pain. See how powerful your mind is?

SOLUTIONS

In moving toward your pain with the will to conquer it, your mind and body can be as powerful as the medication, but without any side effects. In part 3, you will learn how to let go of stress, and in part 4, you will learn both acute and preventative touch therapies.

Although medication advice is beyond the scope of this book, a simple analgesic or a cup of coffee or tea can occasionally be a useful adjunct, especially when you are first learning headache touch therapy. I sometimes take a Tylenol or two to boost the Mundo Method if I get a rare migraine, but I can't always take it because appetite loss is one of my symptoms, and the pill might not stay down on an empty stomach.

Instead of pharmaceuticals, some migraineurs find these herbs, supplements, and remedies helpful for prevention: butterbur, feverfew, magnesium, vitamin B_2 (riboflavin),[6] CoQ10, omega-3 fatty acids, magnesium and feverfew formulations, and homeopathic remedies. Others try cannabis products, where legal (although for some people, cannabis can be a trigger).

Medical electronics companies are researching and introducing noninvasive neuromodulation devices as alternatives to medication therapies for migraine. Currently, three are FDA-approved for prevention; they apply direct current or magnetic stimulation to the head to produce changes in the brain.[7]

If you are committed to getting off your meds, the preventive and relief therapies, exercises, advice, and guidelines imparted in this book are designed to support you. By gradually incorporating holistic, hands-on somatic self-care practices, you won't need medications or feel fearful of living without them. In other words, you can feel better without medications or a device.

Hormonal Triggers

Ladies: Blame your hormones! (Oh, how I wish I were kidding.)

When we consider that two-thirds of migraine sufferers are female (21–22 million women compared to 7 million men in the United States)[8] and that their reproductive hormones affect them throughout their lives, it makes sense that hormones would be a factor in migraines. Another clue: migraine in women is most prevalent during their peak reproductive years, especially from the twenties to the early fifties.

In her informative, in-depth book *The Woman's Guide to Managing Migraine*, women's headache specialist and board-certified family physician Susan Hutchinson explains that women are most likely to get migraine when their hormone levels change, especially estrogen. Estrogen levels drop before each period, during ovulation, after giving birth, during perimenopause, at the tail end of an estrogen patch, after surgical menopause, and during the placebo week of birth control pills, the birth control vaginal ring, and the birth control patch.[9]

Hormonal triggers are somewhat predictable during certain life stages. A benign headache can arise during and after giving birth, due not only to the hormonal changes during birthing but also to medication, medical procedures, physical strain, and lack of food and caffeine. Some women with a history of migraine find relief in the second and third trimesters of pregnancy, when estrogen levels are high, as well as during subsequent months of breast-feeding, when ovulation is dormant. Migraine frequency decreases in two-thirds of women after physiologic menopause but only in one-third of women after surgical removal of their ovaries.[10]

Menstrual Migraine

In an estimated 60 percent of women with migraine in the United States (or about 13 million), there is a connection to their hormonal cycles. An estimated 14 percent have purely *menstrual migraine*, meaning onset only occurs between two days before and three days into their periods. The majority of women with menstrual migraine also have *menstrual-related migraine*, which means they get menstrual migraine plus have episodes at other times during the month. In 40 percent of women with migraine, there appears to be no connection to their cycles.[11]

Hormone therapies for migraine are a mixed bag; for each individual case, a protocol might help, hurt, or have no effect. Doctors often prescribe birth control and hormone replacement therapy to decrease migraine frequency, but it can make them worse. To prevent pregnancy, birth control pills contain more estrogen than is naturally present in the body, but the estrogen drop in the placebo week is larger than it would be normally, creating more vulnerability to migraine. Timed-release birth control pills, patches, and intra-uterine devices (IUDs) are very long acting, which can be a burden and a blessing, depending on how one's migraines are affected.[12]

Dr. Hutchinson advises that the goal of managing menstrual migraine is to even out estrogen levels, so the cyclical drops are less extreme. She cites a broad range of protocols for working with birth control, hormone replacement, and add-back estrogen.[13]

Comorbidity

Women with migraine — as compared to the general female population — are more likely to have certain other conditions in addition. The term for this is *comorbidity*, meaning people have two (or more) conditions that could potentially be related. For migraine, these conditions are anxiety, depression, premenstrual syndrome (PMS) and premenstrual dysphoric disorder (PMDD), history of sexual trauma, fibromyalgia, sleep disturbances, endometriosis, and irritable bowel syndrome.[14] Many of my headache clients have suffered from some of these conditions and so they carry an additional physical and emotional burden, making resolution more complicated (but not impossible). If you are being treated with medication for comorbid conditions, check for headache as a side effect.

Solutions

Whether you are taking hormones for migraine, for birth control, or as hormone replacement therapy, if you have migraine, success will often require a process of experimenting, with your practitioner, to find the right hormonal formulation and dosage for your needs that also keeps your episodes at bay. Hormones are powerful regulators on multiple levels, and how your body responds is totally individual.

Licensed acupuncturists, doctors of Oriental medicine (OMD), naturopathic and homeopathic doctors, registered dietitians, herbalists, and some OB/GYNs can provide natural, holistic solutions for regulating hormone levels.

As I learned from my own menstrual migraines and perimenopause, herbs and supplements can nicely complement lifestyle, meditative, dietary, and hands-on practices. The ones that worked in my case were dong quai, black cohosh, Siberian ginseng, DHEA, and qi tonics prescribed by my acupuncturist/herbalist. Keeping my life in healthy balance made me less vulnerable to changing hormone levels.

9   Diet for Migraine Prevention

*T*his chapter contains a complete plan for preventing migraine with diet. For twenty-five years, this plan has transformed the lives of innumerable migraine sufferers who have followed the Mundo Program.

Diet is essential to migraine management, but not in the ways you might expect. Rodolfo Low was a chemist, professor, Ford Foundation advisor, and migraine sufferer. In *Victory over Migraine: The Breakthrough Study That Explains What Causes It and How It Can Be Completely Prevented through Diet*, he presented the findings of his twenty-two years of clinical research.[1] Drawing a connection between insulin levels and migraine, he concluded that patients can eliminate their migraines altogether by better managing their blood sugar levels, for which he advised a hypoglycemic diet.

This diet boils down to a simple formula: Eat more protein more often, and eat fewer simple carbs. Based on these ideas, this chapter explains what it means when people regularly wake up with headaches, why it's important to eat protein in the morning, and what's wrong with carb breakfasts, energy bars, and sweet snacks.

Migraine and Low Blood Sugar

In 1990, I found Low's little red book in a used bookstore. Since then, the author's ideas have formed the basis of my approach to a diet that has prevented more migraines than almost anything else — and it's shockingly simple!

Dr. Low, a migraine sufferer since childhood, noticed a pattern about his and others' migraine episodes and began doing clinical research to investigate his hypothesis: when migraine-prone people consume foods containing simple carbohydrates, such as refined sugars, corn syrup, fructose, and maltose, they get migraine attacks. (He always got them after a day spent at the movies consuming lots of candy.) For over two decades, Dr. Low analyzed how sugar, or glucose, is metabolized in patients who are prone to migraine. It's complicated (and of course the science is always advancing), but in a laywoman's vastly simplified terms, here's the story:

All the food we eat is metabolized, or broken down, into a sugar called *glucose*, which is then processed by the liver before it enters the bloodstream. Some of the glucose is used immediately, and some is stored as fat so it can be accessed later. When the pancreas is overactive (a condition called *hyperinsulinemia*), it secretes too much insulin, the hormone that controls the amount of sugar in the blood. As a result, too much sugar is eaten up by the excess insulin, resulting in a condition called *hypoglycemia*, or low blood sugar.

Hypoglycemia reduces the body's energy. In order to boost energy, the adrenal glands release the "speedy" hormones, adrenaline and catecholamine. These energy boosters, which are also produced in response to stress, cause blood vessels to constrict, which causes release of lipids called prostaglandins, involved in dilation and inflammation of blood vessels in your head. The dilated blood vessels impinge upon surrounding nerves, sending signals to your brain stem and brain and…now you've got migraine.

Low found that people with migraine are different than those with normal pancreatic functioning in that their blood sugar levels begin lower, rise higher, and end lower. When Low gave migraineurs a glucose tolerance test, he noticed a rapid rise pattern of their blood sugar levels and extended below-average levels after the blood sugar dropped. Low claimed that this characteristic pattern was missed in typical glucose tolerance tests, which took blood samples at half- to one-hour intervals. However, instead of suggesting that migraineurs take the test following his fifteen-minute sampling protocol to learn if their migraines were due to hypoglycemia, Low suggested that they could simply change their dietary habits and *prevent* their migraines.

What Is a Hypoglycemic Diet?

You'd think that in order to increase blood sugar levels, you should eat more sugar, right? Some doctors used to think that was true and suggested it to their patients, but in fact, it's just the opposite.

Patients could eliminate their migraine episodes completely, Low advised, by managing their blood sugar levels with a hypoglycemic diet, consisting of balanced meals of protein, natural carbohydrates, vegetables, and fruits in six small meals, or three meals and three snacks per day. His diet emphasized protein and timing, and suggested smaller meals and snacks to avoid feeling too full to eat every two to three hours.

If you are concerned that eating so frequently will cause weight gain, know that I have observed just the opposite in my clients. If anything, they report losing weight on this diet. This outcome could be due to a combination of increased metabolism, without the extreme rises and dips in blood sugar and energy, and increased activity levels due to feeling better. When your blood sugar is low, your body produces stress hormones to boost your energy, wreaking havoc on your neuroendocrine system. This sort of stress causes you to store fat and crave simple sugars and carbohydrates. When you switch to a healthy diet on a regular schedule, your body no longer gets signals that indicate you might be starving, so you store less fat.

Early Protein

"Early protein" is my shorthand reminder to eat protein first thing in the morning, which is crucial if you wake up with migraines. By eating early protein, you will crave fewer sweets and simple carbohydrates throughout your day and have more consistent energy.

What do people eat for breakfast in the United States? Our nation has become a country of grab-and-go, carb-loaded breakfasts: a bagel and cream cheese; a muffin, Danish, or pastry; a bowlful of sugar-sweetened cereal, granola, or yogurt; juice, coffee, tea, soda, or a sweet espresso drink. Contrast that with Mexico, Central and South America, and the Caribbean, where a traditional breakfast is either eggs, corn tortillas with beans, rice and beans, or bread with cheese and ham, and, of course, café con leche. In Europe, breakfast is eggs, a pastry, or bread with cheese, and café au lait, cappuccino, or café latte. In Japan, breakfast starts with miso soup, followed by rice with tofu, maybe some seafood, a serving of vegetables, and tea.

Why is a carb-loaded breakfast bad for migraineurs? When you sleep, your pancreas is still working, secreting insulin that is ready and waiting to metabolize your breakfast. A muffin or a bagel, which contains about three hundred fifty calories and fifty to sixty grams of carbohydrates — or the equivalent of almost four slices of bread — makes your blood sugar rise and drop rapidly, followed by adrenal and neurovascular responses that trigger migraine.

A lox and bagel story: A student in my class was a busy radiologist who had a long commute, early hospital hours, and a new baby.

Of course, he was sleep deprived and usually skipped breakfast or had just a bagel and cream cheese. Migraines plagued him daily and weighed down his morale. When I asked if he liked lox, a smoked salmon rich in protein and omega-3 fatty acids, he replied that he loved it, so I suggested that he add it to his bagel and cream cheese. To his surprise and delight, eating early protein completely eliminated his episodes — despite his ongoing stressful routine and disrupted sleep. Yes, the bagel was the delivery system, but the lox made all the difference, and he did fine with it. And that was him. Everyone is different, and I encourage you to experiment to find the early protein foods you like.

More Than Diet

Here's where the Mundo Program diverges from Dr. Low's advice. Instead of completely eliminating sugars, this program allows for a little bit of sugar, depending on individual tolerances and the right timing.

Enjoyment — of food, eating, and dining — is an important part of life. After all, the goal is to eliminate your migraines, not your foods. Why needlessly deprive yourself of something that doesn't harm you? If you pay careful attention to cause and effect, you will decipher your patterns and figure out what, if anything, to eliminate or change. For example, if you eat a healthy meal with plenty of protein, you can probably enjoy a dessert with no problem, as long as you don't go overboard (and have eaten protein throughout the day).

That is why your Headache Diary is such an important tool. You will see the effects of potential triggers right before your eyes, laid out day by day, and you'll come to understand how the timing of what you eat, combined with everything else, affects you.

Speaking of "everything else": this is a somatic program, where you work with your entire self. So although your diet is significant in solving your migraine mystery, it is only a part of the story. The tension in your head, neck, and shoulders, how you breathe and use your body, how you respond to stress and feel about your life, your emotional history — you are all of that, and it all plays a role.

Healthy Diet Guidelines

The following Healthy Diet Guidelines provide a framework for what to eat and when, and foods to watch out for or avoid. It also prepares you to track your diet in chapter 10.

1. KEEP A DAILY RECORD.
- Record what and when you eat each day.
- Keeping a daily record is the best way to discover your triggers and see if you are eating well and often enough to maintain stable blood sugar levels, a key to staving off migraine.

2. EAT EVERY TWO TO THREE HOURS.
- Eat three meals and three snacks per day, or six small meals.
- Follow this meal schedule: breakfast, snack, lunch, snack, dinner, snack.
- The snacks do not have to be large, just a little something. You can eat smaller meals, if desired, so you won't be too full for snacks in between.

3. BOOST YOUR PROTEIN.
- Include protein in each meal and snack.
- Find ways to incorporate protein into the dishes you prepare, and into your diet overall.
- Protein foods include eggs, dairy, soy, fish, chicken, meat, beans, and nuts.

4. REDUCE THE AMOUNT OF TIME BETWEEN
   WAKING UP AND EATING.

- Eat breakfast as soon as possible after you wake up.
- If you work out first thing in the morning, eat a protein snack or breakfast first.
- Eat breakfast *before* leaving for work or doing any activities — even at home. Do not wait until you are at your desk or your destination, or until you take a break and "finally have time to eat."
- Adapt this guideline to your schedule if your day starts in the afternoon or you work at night. Your day begins whenever you wake up.

5. EAT "EARLY PROTEIN."

- Start your day with protein to boost your blood sugar levels.

6. KICK THE CAFFEINE.

- The amount of combined daily caffeine from coffee, tea, soda, medication, and chocolate adds up. It can transform an occasional headache or migraine into a chronic condition.
- As discussed in chapter 6, caffeine constricts the blood vessels in your head. When it wears off, they dilate and impinge on the nerves surrounding them, triggering a headache or migraine.
- Do not quit caffeine cold turkey! Stair-step down. (Read that again, three more times.) To avoid getting an extended withdrawal headache, do not let your excitement about the potential of eliminating this trigger sway you to kick it all at once. (I emphasize this warning after seeing countless clients get so enthused to learn of the migraine-caffeine connection that they quit cold turkey — despite my admonitions — only to suffer horrible withdrawal migraines.)

- Kick caffeine in stages: Substitute one-quarter of your usual amount with decaf for at least one week. Then substitute one-half of your usual with decaf, for at least one week. Then substitute three-quarters with decaf. Finally, after at least a month, you'll be drinking all decaf. If you get a withdrawal headache during the process, substitute less than a quarter per stage and stay at each plateau longer.
- After kicking caffeine, drink only water, decaf beverages, and herbal tea until you have no more headaches from any cause. Then you can have an occasional small caffeinated coffee or tea, or perhaps even one per day, and see how it affects you. (I didn't include soda or energy drinks due to their high sugar and caffeine content.) Note in the caffeine chart on page 63 that a shot of espresso contains less than half the caffeine found in a cup of brewed coffee.

7. STICK TO A REGULAR MEAL SCHEDULE.
- Do not skip meals or go hungry.
- Sleeping in on weekends or during a vacation can disrupt your regular meal and caffeine schedule.
- If you will be having brunch, eat a little something first thing in the morning. The same thing goes if you are going out for lunch or dinner. Don't "save up" your appetite.
- If you have a meeting, class, or other activity, bring a healthy snack and your water with you.

8. BE AWARE OF SUGARS AND ARTIFICIAL SWEETENERS IN ALL FOODS AND DRINKS.
- Look for sugar content, listed on product labels as *beet sugar, cane sugar, corn syrup, dextrose, fructose, glucose, high-fructose corn syrup, maltose, sucrose,* and *sugar.* Use sparingly and avoid sugars when possible by choosing alternatives.

- *Take note:* Four grams of sugar equals one teaspoon. So, for example, if a half-cup of ice cream has twenty grams of sugar, that's five teaspoons, nearly the daily maximum amount recommended.[2]
- Sugar is added to canned fruit, applesauce, and juices. Instead, have fresh or dried fruit (unsulfured), canned fruit in juice, and unsweetened applesauce and fruit juice (or sweetened with other juices).
- Look for sugar content in savory foods as well, such as tomato, cream, and butter sauces; soup and gravy; condiments like salad dressing, sweet relish, and ketchup; canned vegetables; and frozen vegetables in sauce.
- Low-calorie foods have less fat but often contain more sugar to boost flavor.
- Do not substitute artificial sweeteners, found in many low-calorie products, for sugars. (See chapter 6, page 67.)
- Satisfy your sweet tooth by consuming natural, healthy foods that are slightly sweet, instead of foods with artificial sweeteners.
- Control your sugar intake by preparing your own food — whether it's salad dressing or dessert.

9. Do not consume "stand-alone sweets."

- *Stand-alone sweets* is my term for a high-sugar food, whether that be a piece of candy, cake, or pie, a cookie, cupcake, muffin, pastry, or an energy bar, without a protein partner, such as a meal or a serving of milk.
- Tack sweets (dessert) to the end of a protein meal instead of having them as a snack.
- Skip the energy bar. Check the label: made for quick energy and loaded with carbs, energy bars are like health-food candy bars. Even an energy bar with high protein is not a meal or

a good snack for a migraine sufferer because it spikes blood sugar levels.

- Skip sweet smoothies, especially for breakfast, and even those with added protein.

- If you want a cookie, choose one that's less sweet, perhaps without icing or filling, like a plain shortbread, galette, biscotti, breakfast biscuit, or fruit juice–sweetened cookie.

- Have your sweet with milk (cow, soy, rice, almond, hemp, or goat). *Note:* Rice and almond milk have one to three grams of protein, and soy and cow milk have seven to eight grams of protein per serving.

- Ice cream in moderation can be okay without added coatings, sugary goodies, candies, swirls, or preservatives. Keep it simple. Watch out for chocolate if it is one of your triggers.

- Exercise portion control. One or two cookies might not bother you, but three or more might, even with protein.

10. Opt for natural carbohydrates.

- Eat foods rich in natural carbohydrates along with protein foods — the key word here being *natural* — such as whole grains, sweet potatoes, potatoes, and pasta. Balanced meals will even out your blood sugar levels and help you digest the protein.

- Unrefined whole grains and flours, such as 100 percent whole wheat, brown rice, steel-cut oats, buckwheat, and corn, contain healthy nutrients and fiber, which are separated out in refined versions.

- Choose cereals that are free of added sugars or lightly sweetened with honey or fruit juice.

- Sometimes your stomach wants the comfort of white basmati rice served with butter and nutritional yeast, or a French baguette with butter. It's okay to mix it up, in moderation, depending on your mood and tummy.

11. EAT FOODS RICH IN OMEGA-3 FATTY ACIDS.

- Unsaturated fats called omega-3 fatty acids, sourced from animals and plants, are an essential part of the human diet.

- Omega-3 is beneficial for people with migraines because it tones and relaxes smooth muscle tissue, the type that makes up the cardiovascular system, including blood vessels in your head related to migraine.

- The so-called fatty fishes, rich in omega-3, include (from high to low content) herring, sardines, mackerel, salmon, halibut, tuna, swordfish, greenshell/green-lipped mussels, tilefish, canned tuna, pollock, caviar, and oysters.

- Omega-3 is abundant in eggs, and grass-fed chickens produce eggs with more of it. Similarly, grass-fed beef has higher omega-3 content than grain- and corn-fed beef.

- Nut and seed sources of omega-3 include flaxseeds and flaxseed oil, canola oil, soybeans, soybean oil, chia seeds, walnuts, and walnut oil.

- The wild green purslane, considered a pesky weed by many gardeners, is the highest source of omega-3 of any leafy green vegetable and is also high in vitamins E and C.

- Omega-3, alone or in combination with omega-6 fatty acids, can be bought in supplement form, but it is better to consume it in food, which provides other nutrients.

- The U.S. Department of Agriculture advises eating foods rich in omega-3 fatty acids two times per week.

12. EAT MAGNESIUM-RICH FOODS.

- Magnesium is an essential mineral that helps control smooth muscle tissue tone and many important chemical reactions in the body. It also helps prevent migraine.

- The following foods are rich in magnesium: dark leafy greens, pumpkin and sesame seeds, Brazil nuts, pine nuts, almonds, pecans, walnuts, pollock, mackerel, tuna, white beans, French beans, kidney beans, pinto beans, black-eyed peas, chickpeas, lentils, brown rice, quinoa, millet, and bulgur.

- Avocado, yogurt, goat cheese, bananas, dried figs, prunes, apricots, dates, and raisins are also magnesium rich. *Note: Many of these foods also contain amines, which can be triggers for some migraineurs.*

- Dark chocolate also contains magnesium, but put it in the "migraine mixed-bag" category because it is also a trigger for some people.

13. EAT A VARIETY OF PRODUCE.

- Eating a variety of fresh vegetables and fruits is essential for good nutrition.

- In hot summer months, eat fresh salads and uncooked fruits and vegetables, which are cooling.

- In cold autumn and winter months, lightly steam, sauté, or bake vegetables and make soups to keep your system heated, hearty, and less susceptible to colds, flu, and upper body tightness.

- In winter, balance fresh produce with dried, canned, baked, or frozen, depending on availability. Purchase canned products packaged in bottles or BPA-free cans. By canning or freezing your own, you can control the ingredients.

- Beware of dried fruits preserved with sulfites, sulfates, or sulfur dioxide. These preservatives help fruit retain its color (like those bright-orange apricots!) but can trigger a migraine.

14. DRINK LOTS OF WATER.

- Drink at least two quarts or liters of pure water per day. Tea, coffee, juice, milk, and soda do not count in that calculation.

- Water keeps your body hydrated, aids with digestion, and is just as necessary during winter as summer. Mild dehydration can make you feel tired and have low energy. Don't ignore your thirst or wait until you feel thirsty.
- Use a water bottle made of stainless steel, glass, or BPA-free plastic.
- If you are not used to water or do not like drinking it, get a bottle with a pull-up spout. You can ingest more easily by sucking (the first way we learn to eat) than by sipping.
- Drink a sixteen-ounce glass of water first thing in the morning. Use large glasses instead of small ones to increase your water intake.
- Keep a water bottle or tall glass of water next to your desk.
- Carry water with you wherever you go — in your car, running errands, to work, meetings, classes, recreational activities, workouts. A ten-minute errand can easily turn into an hour or two, and without your water, you will be "going thirsty."
- Find water that you like. If you do not like the taste of water, you can develop a palate for it; just as you prefer one brand of juice, soda, coffee, or tea over another, experiment to find the water you like. I prefer distilled or reverse-osmosis and carbon-purified water over mineral water because it tastes sweeter to me. The point is, I like it so I drink more.
- Drink water throughout your day. Try not to guzzle it all at once when you realize you are thirsty, especially at night, when drinking too much might make you wake up to use the bathroom. Pace yourself.
- "If you feel thirsty, you are already dehydrated." Have you heard that claim? Well, it's got a point. If you are not always aware of, or you ignore, your body's cues, then yes,

by the time you become aware of your thirst you might be dehydrated.

- Research your best options for clean, safe drinking water. Technology to detect and combat pollutants is always advancing, and in some areas you can drink the tap water unfiltered. Filtered options include carbon-filtered pitchers, filtered faucet attachments to remove chlorine and other chemicals that appear in the water or from old pipes, and bottle delivery.

15. BECOME A LABEL (AND MENU) CHECKER.

- Check "Nutrition Facts" labels and "Ingredients" lists when food shopping. Ingredients are listed in descending order, with the largest quantity first.
- Beware of items with sugar listed first, second, or third, which usually means there is a lot.
- When dining out or ordering takeout, read or ask about ingredients in menu items or prepared foods. Many migraineurs are afraid of going out to eat because they've had bad experiences in the past. They prefer cooking at home rather than suffering the consequences of a hidden ingredient.
- Order more simply prepared foods to control for unknown, potentially triggering ingredients.
- Opt for oil-and-vinegar shakers instead of premade dressing, which can contain preservatives.
- Ask for the gravy, sauce, or dressing on the side so you can control the portion or opt to not eat it.
- Avoid salad bars, which often use preservatives to keep lettuce and cucumbers crisp. Make sure ingredients are preservative-free, or get a salad made-to-order.
- Ask nicely about ingredients. Have you seen comedy skits poke fun at picky diners who ask about every single

ingredient, making requests for this and that to be left out? Finicky diners can be amusing, or annoying, but when a trigger can make you sick for days, you owe it to yourself, and anyone else your migraine might affect, to inquire. Ask about ingredients. People will understand, especially if you are gracious and kind about it.

16. AVOID TRIGGER FOODS.

- Keep a Headache Diary to discover and avoid your food triggers (see chapter 10). You can learn a lot by looking for cause and effect.
- When you discover your triggers, you don't have to restrict your diet unnecessarily or go through the process of an elimination diet.

17. PRACTICE THESE HEALTHY EATING TIPS.

- Eat a balanced diet of about 20 to 30 percent protein, 30 percent fat, including seeds and nuts, and 40 to 50 percent carbohydrates, including most fruits, vegetables, grains, and beans.
- Eat about forty grams of protein per day. Athletes might need to eat more. In cases of kidney disease, acute infection, or recovery from an injury, eat less. (Consult your physician or a registered dietitian.)
- Choose in-season, locally grown produce. During the off-season, frozen foods, which have been picked at peak ripeness and are then flash-frozen, are a good alternative.
- Lightly steam or sauté vegetables to retain their nutrients.
- Buy organic when possible to avoid hormones, antibiotics, pesticides, and fungicides.
- Consume fish, free-range poultry, and vegetable protein, such as soybeans, tofu, tempeh (a cultured soybean cake), and black beans, as alternatives to red meat.

18. Be prepared.

- Set aside the time needed to plan, shop for, prepare, and eat healthy meals and snacks, even when you're away from home. Be prepared, so you don't end up grabbing what might be quick but unhealthy.

19. Enjoy your food.

- As a migraine sufferer, you might be used to focusing more on what to avoid than on what you can enjoy. If you have curbed your diet over time based on a general triggers list, perhaps you have forgotten the satisfaction of a balanced diet.
- Here's an illustration of what I mean: One of my clients had stopped eating bananas, which she loved, because they were on a triggers list. But she felt deprived. Bananas have fiber, potassium, and vitamins B and C, and they are low in calories. While keeping her Headache Diary, she tried a banana and found that bananas were not her trigger after all, so she added them back into her diet. With this simple change, she felt more like a normal person who didn't have to be so picky about her food choices. Overall, it lightened her mood and eased her stress because she could have something enjoyable and nourishing.
- Find headache-healthy foods you like, and do not deprive yourself needlessly. Keeping a Headache Diary will help you identify your personal triggers rather than eliminating everything that is on a list. Curb only those foods that are harmful for you. I want you to savor life to the fullest.

Headache-Healthy Diet Suggestions

Now that you know the Healthy Diet Guidelines, the following listing of menu and food ideas will assist you in making good choices throughout your day. Use these suggestions as a jumping-off point to build your own headache-healthy diet and menu plans. Have at least one food from each group — protein, carbohydrate (this can be omitted if you wish), fruit/vegetable, and beverage — per meal.

Breakfast

Protein: eggs, unsweetened yogurt, Greek yogurt, scrambled tofu, lox and cream cheese, cottage cheese, farmer's cheese, beans, tempeh, cheddar (if not sensitive to it) and other cheeses, nuts/nut butter (walnuts, almonds, pecans, cashews, peanuts), breakfast sausage or bacon (preservative-free) or vegetarian sausage/bacon

- Milk, yogurt, and cheese products can be made from cow, goat, soy, hemp, almond, cashew, and rice milk. Cow, goat, soy, and hemp milk contain five to eight grams of protein, and almond, cashew, and rice milk contain one to three grams, per eight-ounce serving.
- *Note:* Greek-style yogurt contains twice as much protein as regular. Full-fat and low-fat yogurt are preferable to non-fat because the fat content digests more slowly, which is better for blood sugar levels. Avoid yogurt sweetened with high-fructose corn syrup and fruit syrup.

Carbohydrate: whole-grain toast, bagel or English muffin, cold cereal or granola, hot cereal with salt and butter or nut butter, biscuits, whole-grain muffin sweetened with fruit juice, pancakes or whole-grain waffles, rice, tortillas (flour or corn)

Fruit/vegetable: fresh, frozen, or dried fruit (use banana, berries, peaches, nectarines, or raisins to sweeten cereal), fruit spread, fruit compote, sliced tomato, avocado, vegetables (in omelet or tofu), salsa

Beverage: water, decaf or herbal coffee or tea, seltzer / club soda, vegetable or fruit juice without added sugar

How to Combine Food Groups for Breakfast
The possibilities are endless!

- Eggs, scrambled or soft-boiled, with toast and butter or cream cheese; sliced tomato
- Avocado toast
- Sliced fruit topped with plain yogurt, drizzled with honey, sprinkled with nuts and flaxseed meal. Serve with a slice of whole-grain toast with butter, nut butter, or smashed avocado
- Waffle topped with strawberries, yogurt, drizzle of maple syrup or honey; breakfast sausage
- An orange, a tangerine, or a half grapefruit; toasted English muffin or whole-grain bread with butter and a dab of jam or fruit spread; cottage cheese
- Leftovers for breakfast: for example, a taco or burrito made with beans or chicken, lettuce, tomato, avocado, yogurt, cheese, and salsa
- Half bagel, mini bagel, or scooped-out whole bagel with lox, cream cheese, sliced tomato, and red onion

Lunch and Dinner

Lunch is so nice, you can have it twice! Not really. But yes, lunch and dinner have the same choices here. Many of us are creatures of habit; we eat the same thing every day for a particular meal. Looking at the choices for lunch and dinner together allows you to think ahead about what you would like for each and balance out what you eat each day. Mix it up. Looking at a variety of choices might spark something new for you.

Protein: tuna, egg, tofu, cheese (cottage, cheddar, Swiss, jack, Havarti, provolone, mozzarella), grilled or baked fish/seafood, chicken, turkey, beef, beans (soy, black, chickpeas, pinto, red, black-eyed peas, lentils), veggie burger, tempeh, falafel, hummus, nut butter, protein-based chili, stew, soup

Carbohydrate: whole-grain bread or crackers, tortilla, pita, corn bread, pasta, tabbouleh, rice, quinoa, bulgur, couscous, millet, buckwheat, barley, potato, sweet potato

Fruit/vegetable: lettuce, arugula, salad greens, avocado, veggies — steamed, stir-fried, or baked (broccoli, kale, Swiss chard, collards, cauliflower, cabbage, bok choy, mustard greens, turnips, rutabaga, kohlrabi, radish, green beans, peas, carrots, parsnips, winter squash, summer squash, peppers, eggplant, tomato), vegetable-based soup, tomato sauce, fruit (bananas, apples, pears, berries, pineapple, peaches, apricots, nectarines, pluots, melon, grapes, cherries, citrus, mango, papaya)

Beverage: water, decaf coffee or tea, herbal tea, fruit or vegetable juice, fruit juice–sweetened soda, juice mixed with soda water or seltzer (make your own to taste with grape, apple, cherry, or orange juice, or cranberry juice sweetened with other juices)

How to Combine Food Groups for Lunch/Dinner

My dietitian mom used to make these Eastern European–influenced, protein-packed dishes. What healthy dishes you were raised on?

- Farmer's chop suey: cottage cheese and sour cream or plain yogurt, mixed with chopped cucumber, tomato, green pepper, green onion, and radish. This dish is refreshing in summer, served with rye bread and butter or whole-grain crackers.
- Extra-wide egg noodles, cooked and tossed with butter and salt, topped with a dollop of cottage cheese. Serve with

steamed broccoli, butter, and salt — and for extra protein, salmon croquettes.

- Salmon or tofu loaf or croquettes, meatloaf or turkey meatloaf, meatballs (use turkey, pork, textured vegetable protein, or tofu). Serve one of these as a main dish, adding roasted or steamed vegetables and mashed potatoes.

- Frittata, quiche, or omelet made with your choice of cheese, vegetables, and other protein, served with a green salad and a piece of crusty sourdough bread with butter

Does this array of possibilities give you some ideas about how to expand your menu and choices? Combine foods to make a sandwich, burrito, pita sandwich, stir-fry, pasta and protein dish, soup, salad, or stew. How about sushi — whether fish or vegetarian? It contains protein, vegetables, and rice. Just check for preservatives if you don't make it yourself.

Many clients and students who first come into my practice or join a class aren't clear on what a healthy diet looks like. Their diet is typically something like this: smoothie for breakfast (basically carbs with a little protein), salad for lunch (with little or no protein), and then, finally, protein at dinner (making this the first substantial protein of the day). They think this diet is healthy because it's low calorie and contains fruit and vegetables, and they are surprised to learn it's not a great diet for migraineurs. As emphasized in this chapter, eating protein meals and snacks *throughout* the day stabilizes blood sugar levels. Switching to the diet detailed in this chapter makes all the difference.

Snacks and Desserts

The list below offers a variety of healthy choices to keep you from going astray. Remember to pair your snack with protein unless protein is already a main ingredient. Use these suggestions to spark your imagination, then go online, read cookbooks, and watch cooking shows for more ideas.

Snacks can be savory or sweet. For savory items, like chips, pop-corn, crackers, and popped chips, check for artificial flavorings, seasonings, food dyes, and preservatives — just as you would for sweets. For sweet baked goods and frozen treats, omit those with icing, sweet filling, chocolate or yogurt chips, candy, candied fruit, sugary swirl add-ins, and sweet toppings. Try fruit juice–sweetened cookies, muffins, and frozen goods. You can best control for sugars by making your own.

Monitor quantity. Have a small portion of a sweet snack — one or two cookies, a half of a "regular-size" item, or a mini-muffin. Two tablespoons of chocolate ice cream (milk is protein) might be okay for you, but half a cup or a cup might trigger your migraine. If any amount of chocolate triggers you, perhaps vanilla or another flavor won't.

Breads: pretzels, crackers (crunchy multigrain, wheat, rye, or rice crackers, or water crackers), tortilla (corn or flour, heated), whole-grain toast. Serve with dip (such as hummus, cottage cheese, blended tofu dip, salsa, or guacamole), hard cheese or goat cheese, or top with nut butter and a drizzle of honey or sliced banana. A pizza slice combines three food groups!

Chips: corn, pita, bagel, corn and bean, potato, vegetable. Try baked or reduced-fat chips. Serve with salsa, guacamole, or bean dip.

Cookies, bars, muffins, quick breads: cookie (biscotti, zwieback, animal crackers, graham crackers, digestive biscuit), granola bar, whole-grain fruit bar, nutrition bar, muffin, scone, quick bread (ba-nana, zucchini, pumpkin). Try low-sugar or fruit juice–sweetened items with added fruit and nuts.

Frozen treats: frozen fruit (try blueberries, raspberries, strawberries, mangoes, grapes, peaches); ice cream, gelato, or frozen yogurt, with natural toppings like fresh fruit or nuts; frozen fruit bars sweetened with juices (make your own in popsicle or ice-cube trays)

Fruit: dried fruit, unsulfured (raisins, dates, figs, prunes, apricots, apples, peaches — plain or with nuts); fresh fruit with cottage cheese or plain yogurt, drizzle of honey; apple or banana served with nut butter (peanut, almond, cashew, soy); applesauce, unsweetened; fruit compote made from dried prunes, pears, peaches, and/or apricots and served with cottage cheese, yogurt, or milk; canned fruit in fruit juice

Juice: vegetable, fruit, or combined (unsweetened fresh, bottled, or canned)

Milk: cow, soy, goat, almond, cashew, rice, hemp, cold or warm (can add honey and nutmeg)

Milk and cold cereal or granola: naturally sweetened with fresh or dried fruit

Nuts: walnuts, almonds, pecans, cashews, hazelnuts, Brazil nuts, filberts; pair with raisins, dates

Popcorn: pop your own; add salt, butter, nutritional yeast (see vegetarian section below)

Smoothie: fresh or frozen berries, banana, peaches, your choice of milk. Try adding kale, carrots, other veggies.

Trail mix: Try making your own. If store-bought, avoid candied fruit and candy chips.

Veggies: carrot and celery sticks; green, red, yellow, and orange pepper strips; cherry tomatoes; broccoli and cauliflower florets. Serve with hummus, goat cheese, vegetable or onion dip (check for MSG), cottage cheese, blended tofu dip.

Can you have just one? Remember, everything in moderation. That's why tracking is so important: Each person's "moderation" is as different as each person's body. A couple of chocolate chip cookies or an energy bar might have zero effect on someone else but be dangerous for you. If you can't refrain from eating the whole row or package of cookies, it's best to not have them around — or to choose an option that's less sweet. If you find yourself bingeing and then suffering from a migraine the following day, it's time to let that snack go and find another.

Vegetarians Must Eat Beans

When people switch to a vegetarian or vegan diet, they forgo animal products for fruits, vegetables, grains, nuts, and seeds. However, these foods alone do not supply enough daily protein, and limiting yourself to these categories might result in weakness, fatigue, nutritional deficiency, and dissatisfaction with the diet — not to mention migraine. This is why some people who have tried vegetarianism often return to eating meat, reporting disappointedly that their experiment was a failure.

Here's the key: Vegetarians and vegans must eat beans! People need about forty grams of protein per day, and if you don't eat meat you need to get that protein in the form of beans. Soybeans (whether as whole beans, soy milk, tofu, or tempeh), which are a complete protein, have the highest protein value, followed by black beans and chickpeas. When black beans are combined with rice, and pinto beans are combined with corn, they also make a complete protein. Vegans and vegetarians must supplement with vitamin B_{12}, which is an essential nutrient not contained in vegetables or beans.

If they want, vegetarians can also get added protein from dairy and eggs, called *lacto-ovo*. Some people do not eat red meat, pork, or poultry but occasionally eat fish, so they are not technically vegetarians or vegans; they are *pescatarians*. If they have fish only occasionally, they still need to eat beans in order to get sufficient protein.

Vegetarian and vegan versions of products usually made from meat, poultry, and dairy, such as hot dogs, burgers, luncheon meats, and cheese, are made from a base of tofu, soy, wheat gluten, nuts, legumes, veggies, hemp, grains, or dairy (vegetarian items may include milk, eggs, and cheese). These alternatives are commonly carried in grocery and health food stores. You can pick and choose the varieties and brands you like of these quick and easy sources of protein. However, whole beans, tofu, and tempeh generally provide higher-quality protein than these processed foods.

Do you know about nutritional yeast? Sometimes called *large-flake* nutritional yeast (or *nut yeast*, for short), nutritional yeast is a by-product of the molasses-making process; it is *not* brewer's yeast or baking yeast. It has a cheese-like flavor and can be sprinkled on popcorn, cooked vegetables, rice, beans, tofu, and tempeh, and added to salad dressing, sauces, gravies, and soups. It contains all the essential amino acids, making it a tasty, healthy addition to vegan diets.[3] Health food stores usually carry it prepackaged or in the bulk bin section. You might have to ask a knowledgeable staff person to find or order it for you. Store your nut yeast away from light in a covered, opaque container, so the nutrients do not degrade.

One of The Farm community's favorite meals was hand-rolled flour tortillas filled with pressure-cooked soybeans and topped with finely chopped onions, lettuce, tomato salsa, and nutritional yeast. Yum! (To be digestible, soybeans must be cooked until they are as soft as butter — meaning when you press a bean between your tongue and your upper palate, it melts.)[4]

What's on Your Plate?

Nutritional standards and dietary ideas and trends change with the times, shaped by medical and scientific research. The grain-heavy "food pyramid" of my childhood, depicting U.S. Department of Agriculture nutritional guidelines, has been replaced by the more equal distribution of food groups on "My Plate," and no doubt this will change again.

For the past forty years, health-conscious people have followed a low-fat, high-carbohydrate diet for heart health and to lower cholesterol and curb obesity. But recent studies show that good fats, especially olive oil, don't make people fat — sugar does. Sugar consumption in the United States has increased steadily over the past decades, and so have portion sizes.[5] A "small" soda used to be eight ounces; now it's a whopping sixteen or even thirty-two ounces. A quart of soda is now a small!

Another thing we've learned more fully is that carbs are complex sugars: a piece of bread or a tortilla is still a carb — it quickly metabolizes, causing blood sugar swings. The body metabolizes sugar in twenty minutes, carbohydrates in one to two hours. Compare this with protein, which takes five hours, and fats, at seven to eight hours.

This is why full-fat dairy products (like whole or "regular" milk) have regained favor after years of low-fat being advised. For migraineurs who aren't dairy-sensitive, the body can store and use full-fat dairy without the sudden rise and dip in blood sugar produced by the higher lactase (milk sugar) content of reduced-fat products. Whole milk also contains more headache-healthy omega-3 fatty acids. If you are concerned about fat content, eat a smaller portion: have a half-cup instead of a cup of full-fat yogurt, or use 2 percent reduced-fat dairy rather than 1 percent or fat-free.

A high-protein, anti-inflammatory diet with vegetables, fruits, healthy fats, some dairy, and whole grains (usually gluten-free) has been shown to be beneficial in treating autoimmune diseases and inflammation-related conditions. If you are dealing with comorbid conditions, an anti-inflammatory diet might work well for you.[6]

The Mediterranean diet epitomizes the philosophy of "everything in moderation" in terms of food. In successive studies over decades, the Mediterranean diet — made up of vegetables, fruits, fatty fish, whole grains, nuts, legumes, and healthy fats, like olive oil, with some dairy, like yogurt and hard cheeses — has been proven preventative for heart disease, cancer, and other conditions. And it's tasty. The headache-healthy diet in this book is basically that diet minus the wine. Strive to eat balanced meals and snacks and a variety of foods low in saturated fat, sodium, and added sugars, incorporating protein into each.

Diet affects not only migraine but every aspect of your health. Each person is different, and the amount and balance of foods you need depends on your age, physical activity, and health-related factors. For personal nutritional guidance or other health concerns or conditions, especially related to kidney health, diabetes, osteoporosis, or digestion, it's wise to consult with a registered dietitian.

10   Tracking Your Triggers

*I*t's time to track your triggers. This chapter introduces the Headache Diary, an essential tool for discovering your triggers in real life, up close and personal.

If you have kept diaries in the past, you probably recorded your headaches and medications, and perhaps your diet. Our approach is different because it includes all aspects of your life. Instead of recording only your headaches, symptoms, food, and medications, you will be looking at your daily life as a whole — from when you get up to when you go to bed, and into the night, should you have interrupted sleep.

You will record and examine your everyday activities and the self-care practices you learn over the course of the program, noting any changes that result. Tracking in this way will help you determine and address your own specific triggers rather than unnecessarily eliminating those that aren't personally relevant. Feeling miserable *and* deprived is counterproductive to healing!

The Headache Diary is designed with a purpose. First, the entries for each day are chronological, so you can observe what happened exactly as it unfolded. Second, it is formatted in landscape layout so you can see an entire week at a glance, which is fundamental to finding patterns in diet, stress, bodily tension, sleep, and other factors that might add up to your headaches. Consider that your body often has a delayed reaction to what you eat, drink, and do. For example, if you have a glass of wine or piece of chocolate, you'd most likely get a migraine the following day rather than immediately. By looking at the previous day and your whole week, instead of just day by day or trigger by trigger, you will be able to identify the culprits and your recurring patterns more easily — like the migraine you get weekly after a stressful meeting — and a complete picture will begin to form.

The Headache Diary Guidelines listed below act like a packing list of what to include. Each guideline relates to something you need to observe, so you can identify potential triggers. If you get migraines, for example, it is important to know when you wake up, what time you have breakfast or work out, and what you eat. That's because you need to eat protein soon after waking up and before exercising to stabilize blood sugar levels. By recording wake and sleep times, you can see if you are getting enough sleep and what happens when you don't — or if sleep is even a factor for you (it might not be).

Your diary is more than a food journal; it includes your major activities and how you felt about them. You might love your job but have a stressful day if you felt a coworker, boss, client, or customer was unreasonable. Did that stress land on your shoulders, making them tight and primed for a headache? Write it down! Do not take for granted anything that could be a trigger.

Headache Diary Guidelines

- Keep a Headache Diary, with notations for every day, for at least three months.
- Record your entries on the form each day or night, so you will remember the details. It is easy to forget them once you are on to the next day.

- Be totally honest in your diary even if you don't like what you write. Remember, you are a headache detective, looking at your life in order to uncover a mystery, perhaps a treasure trove.

Write down:

1. What time you wake up (use the abbreviation *WU*)
2. What times you eat (including snacks) and drink
3. What you eat and drink (not including water)
4. Total water intake — record it at the bottom of each day's column
5. Physical factors: illness, pain, tension; hormonal changes, menstrual cycle; schedule changes, travel; weather, environment; and more
6. Stressful or outstanding events, occurrences, or interactions
7. Emotions: your thoughts and feelings about events of the day; your mood
8. Self-care practices, physical exercise, and how long you did them: breathing (*BR*), meditation (*MED*), exercise/workout (*WO*), self-massage (*SM*); for example, if you did a breathing exercise for ten minutes and meditated for twenty minutes, you might write *BR 10 min, MED 20 min*
9. Any headaches you get. Again, use an abbreviation (e.g., *migr, TT, mixed*); write *HA* and note the following:

   - Time, pain intensity on a scale of 1 to 10, and duration, such as *HA, 7 AM, #8, 6 hrs*
   - What you do for the headache and how long it takes to work. For example, *SM 30 min, MM* (for "Mundo Method") *1 hr*

10. Any medications, including prescription and nonprescription, that you take, begin taking, or stop taking for headaches or for other conditions

11. Other activities, including work and recreation; major life changes

12. What time you go to sleep

After a few weeks, look at each week's diary in succession and see if any patterns emerge, whether dietary, physical, emotional, postural, environmental, lifestyle, hormonal, or medication related. Read your Headache Diary entries like signs posted along the road of your life, signs that indicate where you are, which way you need to go, and what to adjust in order to stay on your journey to well-being.

Headache Diary Form

Look at the form on the next page.

Enter days of the week and dates across the top. On this form, make the day you start the first day, no matter what day of the week it is. Each day of the week gets a vertical column that goes down the page. The day begins at 6 AM and ends after midnight for chronological tracking. Abbreviate to save space because the column is narrow. For example, you might write *ww toast* for "whole-wheat toast," *Eng muffin* for "English muffin," *cott ch* for "cottage cheese," and so on.

The legend below the form is for quick reference — a shorthand reminder of the Headache Diary Guidelines. Some items are relevant daily, such as what and when you eat and drink. Others you will record less often, such as weather triggers, menstrual cycle, and travel, unless you travel for a living or are on an extended trip. As you learn and add new mind-body practices to your diary, you might notice that your notations about headaches and related symptoms take up less space.

You can, of course, pull up the weekly view calendar on your computer or tablet, but also try printing it out and writing directly on the page. Keeping track on paper allows you to record your day

DAY						
DATE						
6 AM						
12 N						
6 PM						
12 M						
Water						

Record daily:

Time	Diet	Physical Factors	Emotions	Practices/Exercise	Headache (HA)	Other
Wake up (WU)	Foods	Illness, pain, tension	Stress	Breathing (BR)	Type (migr, TT, mixed)	Meds (begin/stop)
Eat/drink	Drinks	Hormonal changes, menstruation	Thoughts	Meditation (MED)	Time started, Length (L: # mins/hrs)	Activities (work, recreation, etc.)
Go to sleep	Water	Schedule changes, travel	Feelings	Exercises, Workout (WO)	Intensity (# on scale of 1–10)	Life changes
		Weather, environment, etc.	Mood	Self-massage (SM)	Remedy (MM, meds, heat/cold)	

even when you don't feel like using a computer, and it makes it easier to compare several weeks or months to search for patterns. Your Headache Diary might be too small to see on your phone or other small screen; you need to be able to easily and chronologically track the details of each day and see your whole week at a glance. That way your diary can support your goal of learning from your life.

What Are You Practicing?

"We are always practicing something," notes author and aikido master George Leonard. There is great value in observing and assessing one's practices as a path to healing. What are you practicing, and how does it add up to your headaches? By diligently recording your practices and then mining your Headache Diary for triggers and patterns, you will come face to face with what you are practicing and how those practices add up.

Lorraine, a young adult with a budding career, took my class through her HMO's health education program. She maintained her busy schedule on a diet of five colas a day and little else and resisted my coaching about it. Then one day in class she announced excitedly that she'd had a breakthrough; the impact of her diet had finally sunk in. After her "aha" moment, she ditched the soda, started making healthy food and lifestyle choices, and guess what? Her headaches disappeared. No magic or mystery, just cause and effect.

Lorraine's view of her life became clear when she decided to look at it in a more serious, methodical way and solve her migraines, instead of holding on to what she *thought* she knew. She had been practicing a cola diet that resulted in rebound headaches from caffeine, sugar, high stress, and lack of real food. When she changed her practices, she got a different result. She could feel the results in her body, and the changes she made were also reflected in her diary. As Gary Player said, "The more I practice, the luckier I get."

The Headache Diary as a Discovery Tool

I get it that diary-keeping can seem like just "one more thing" to do. If you are tempted to view it as an extra chore, remember, it is a tool that will help you. Tracking your daily life is how you can see everything that adds up to your headaches. Then, when you begin to feel better, you will see what produces that improvement too.

After your headache mystery is solved, you can stop keeping your diary. Should your headaches return, you can start journaling again to find out why. Perhaps you momentarily fell off the wagon or didn't know about a hidden ingredient, and you ate or did something that triggered a migraine.

Our office threw a Valentine's Day party with an array of fabulous chocolate candies and cake. I had eaten protein throughout the day, and chocolate is not usually one of my triggers, so I had a few pieces of candy and bites of cake. The next day, I had a horrible migraine that knocked me out, and I concluded that a chemical, food coloring, or preservative in the candy did it.

Sometimes even when we do our best, stuff happens. Don't be hard on yourself. Just look for the connections. One accident does not mean you are backsliding.

What's Happening in Your Body?

Tracking your triggers goes beyond your foods, medications, headaches, and practices. Keeping in mind the Chinese Menu Theory and looking at all parts of your life means paying attention to your mood, your stress, how your body feels that day or that week, and how you felt after a tense interaction.

Where do your feelings live in your body? If we were in-session, I would ask you body-centered questions because I would be looking at you and noticing your breathing, shoulders, language, and mood. As you get more in touch with your body, it will be second nature to check in with yourself in that way. Simply ask yourself "What's happening in my body?" and notice what lights up. If it seems relevant, write it down in your diary in a word or two. We will delve into this more in part 5, "The Deeper Realms of Headache."

What's Your Mood?

When you make big changes in lifestyle and health, your usual patterns get stirred up and challenged, which can produce shifts in mood. Your mood can also shift in response to smaller changes and everyday occurrences, like bad traffic or a sideways glance. Bringing awareness to mood can provide insight into the potentially harmful habits that you have taken for granted.

We all have moods, but instead of us having them, it's easy to feel as if they are having us and there's nothing we can do about it. Identifying your mood is another way to check in with your body and return your attention to the present moment. This process makes mood more visible and thus easier to shift.

During your day, if you notice a particular mood or see that your mood has changed because of something that did or did not happen, check in and add it to your Headache Diary. How did your mood contribute to your headache — or vice versa?

One way to check in with your mood is to try this exercise, which I first practiced in my somatics trainings with Dr. Richard Strozzi-Heckler. I find it comforting.

Mood Check Exercise

What is your mood right now? How do you experience it in your body? To find the answers, simply do this exercise wherever you are. The following example will evoke a couple of moods; then you will learn how to check on your own.

Close your eyes. Imagine that the phone rings, and the caller is someone you really don't want to talk to. What mood comes over you? Do you feel it in your body? If so, what does it feel like? Now imagine instead the caller is someone dear to you, who you really do want to talk to. Describe what that feels like. Your mood changed, and so did your body, right? Your thoughts alone produced those changes without anything else happening.

Check in with your mood throughout the day. By naming and claiming your mood, you have a better chance of managing it. You can name it in one or two words by asking and answering your own question. For example:

Q: What's my mood? A: Happy and excited.

Q: What's my mood? A: Anxious and uptight.

You can also identify the mood *and* describe in a word or two how the mood feels in terms of bodily sensations.

Q: What's my mood? A: Nervous (mood) and sweaty (how it feels in the body).

Q: What's my mood? A: Overjoyed and flushed.

Mood awareness helps produce inner-outer integrity because you are acknowledging what is going on inside yourself rather than ignoring or denying it. It takes practice though, and the hardest part is remembering to do it! You'll notice a prompt for mood in the Headache Diary legend, under "Emotions."

In the process of finding and eliminating your headache triggers and building healthy new practices, you might get jarred, which is a natural reaction when you are trying to make significant lifestyle and behavioral changes. Chances are, you will be examining long-cherished habits, food or beverage choices, or relied-upon therapies, and your mood will be affected. Putting overly high expectations on yourself or others or feeling deprived about what you can or can't eat can also affect your mood.

So be patient with yourself. And right now, simply observe your mood. Notice and be present to how you are and what you feel in the moment — and note it in your diary.

Part Three

Creating Balance through Awareness

11   Breathing In, Breathing Out

We breathe every minute of our lives, but even with all that practice, most of us don't breathe well — or at least effectively and consciously. In this chapter, you will learn why, how, and when to use breathing to calm the stress that contributes to headaches. Zen Buddhist Thích Nhất Hanh describes it beautifully when he says, "Breathing is the best way to stop — to stop unhappiness, agitation, fear, and anger."[1]

Humans cannot survive without breathing for more than a few minutes. Breathing is our birthright and our life force, and yet we take its presence for granted. It happens automatically, so we put it on the back burner. The Hawaiian term for non-natives is *haoles*, meaning "people without breath." This term illustrates how keenly traditional Hawaiian culture is attuned to breathing: Hawaiians could perceive how breath appeared in other people's bodies.

Over the past twenty-five years, I have worked personally and professionally with a wide variety of breathing methods: some for calm, energized centering and others for deep transformation and unwinding of trauma. Countless times I have observed how people breathe — shallow or deep, held or moving — and where the breath is centered and why.

When you practice breathing, you too will start to notice more about it and become able to shift it in real time to address your stress. As you observe the qualities, patterns, sensations, and style of your breathing, you will notice how it reflects each present moment and your overall state of being — and you'll be able to see these things more clearly in others.

How Am I Breathing?

Chronic headache sufferers commonly breathe in stress mode, taking short, rapid, shallow breaths, centered up high in the chest. This stressful breathing creates constant, underlying shoulder, neck, head, and face tension that contributes to ideal headache conditions. Most people are unaware of their shallow breathing, whereas others already know that they have trouble taking comfortable deep breaths.

What do you notice about your breathing? Try this: Take a deep breath. How did you do it? Chances are you took it high in your chest, making it expand and your shoulders rise. That is how most people breathe when stressed, which also makes their shoulders, neck, and chest tight. Breathing high in your body creates a kind of vicious cycle. You get less oxygen, and your breaths get shorter, faster, and shallower in an attempt to get more.

Now, gently place your fingers on the sides of your neck and take another deep breath. Did you feel your neck tighten? Chest breathing creates upper body tension because you are tightening the areas you should be relaxing. On average, humans take twenty thousand breaths per day, so if you are breathing into your chest, that means related muscles and fascia are tightening twenty thousand times per day — just to breathe and without lifting a finger! No wonder your neck and shoulders get tight!

Breathing and the Fight-or-Flight Response

Breathing is directly connected to the fight-or-flight response, the built-in survival mechanism of all animals. This explains why sometimes we cannot relax even when we want to.

Thousands of years ago, our ancestors lived in wilderness habitats. When faced with threats from predators, they had to mobilize quickly, to either fight or flee. When threatened, their bodies responded with an instantaneous, system-wide cascading series of events, starting with alerts in the brain, followed by secretion of "speedy" hormones, increased heart rate, pulse, and blood pressure, blood pushed to the muscles, release of stored energy, and heightened mental alertness. Today most of us don't live in the jungle, threatened by the possibility of being a lion's lunch, but our busy, plugged-in-24/7 lives are stressful and filled with a myriad of activities, opportunities, and responsibilities.

Stress is stress, and even with today's very different stressors, our physiology reacts as if it were fighting for our survival. And now, as never before in history, we are bombarded with images, information, advertising, and opinions that influence our views about body image and health: Girls should be thin, have flat stomachs, and fit into skinny jeans. Boys should be tough and shouldn't cry.

All this stress, all of these overt and covert messages, affect the way we breathe. To many of us, the world feels uncertain and constantly in flux, and our bodies mirror this feeling. Whether it's due to stress, self-consciousness, tight clothing, or peer and societal pressures, holding in the stomach forces the breath into the chest and produces stressful breathing.

Belly Breathing

Have you ever watched babies breathe? They are naturally animated. When they breathe, laugh, and cry, their little bellies round out and then in, while their arms and legs follow along. With their behaviors not yet shaped, they appear to be breathing with their whole bodies.

"Belly breathing" does not mean that your breath goes into your belly; of course, it goes into your lungs. Rather, in belly breathing your belly is relaxed, which allows your diaphragm to drop down and your lungs to take in more air and, thus, more oxygen. Instead of trying to breathe deeper, imagine breathing lower in your body; deeper breathing will occur when you breathe lower.

The diaphragm is a dome-shaped muscle, situated horizontally just below your lungs and attached to your lower ribs, that divides your torso into abdominal and chest cavities. When you take a breath, your lungs fill with air, and the dome flattens, moving toward your abdomen. If your abdomen is tight, your diaphragm cannot drop down, which prevents your lungs from fully expanding. Your body gets less oxygen, which releases stress hormones, creating more stress — and this is how shallow breathing becomes a vicious cycle. Or, as I once heard Gay Hendricks, author of *Conscious Breathing*, put it, "You can't breathe because you can't breathe." The antidote is belly breathing. By breathing lower, into your belly and ribs in addition to your chest, you can shift into a calmer state.

Daily Breathing

Daily Breathing is a set of floor exercises that promotes fuller breathing, mind-body relaxation, energy, and focus. It's an abridged, annotated version of the breathing exercises I learned in the professional training courses of Drs. Gay and Kathlyn Hendricks, whose exhilarating work in this area — which also informs this chapter — introduced me to the transformational world of breathing.[2]

Daily Breathing produces a powerful shift for headache and migraine sufferers, including a steadier mood, less anxiety, and a calm sense of spaciousness. Regular practice helps the small stuff roll off your back, makes you more aware of breath-holding throughout your day, and builds your capacity to take a breath and shift your stress.

Set aside ten minutes in the morning, or five minutes each morning and evening, for the exercises. Record in your diary the time of day and how long you practice. When you're first learning, read through the Preparation and Practice sections before you start, and keep the book open next to you so you can refresh your memory.

Preparation for Daily Breathing

Nonrestrictive clothing is best. Put on yoga pants, sweatpants, leggings, gym shorts, or pajamas. Keep your feet bare or wear socks; no shoes.

1. SET UP YOUR SPACE

- Prepare a comfortable place for lying down on the floor, with enough space around you to extend your legs out straight and your arms fully to each side in a *T* shape.
- Place a rug, yoga mat, pad, or blankets on the floor, so you feel comfortable. (If you're using a sticky yoga mat, cover it with a towel, so you can glide.) Do not lie on a bed or thick foam mattress; they are too soft and bouncy.
- Don't put pillows under your head, neck, or knees.

2. POSITION YOUR BODY

- Lie on your back with your arms by your sides, legs stretched out straight. Bend your knees and slide your feet toward your hips, placing them hip-distance apart (about a foot).
- Give your legs a good base. Here's how to find the optimal support for your legs:

- o Slide your feet farther away from your hips; if your legs feel less stable, that's too far away. Then pull your feet in very close to your hips, and notice how it feels restrictive. That's too close.
- o Now place your feet a comfortable distance between too far away from and too close to your hips. Your legs should feel well supported.

- Recheck that your feet are hip-distance apart with knees open, in line with your hips. If your knees are held together or there is tension between your thighs, your spine will not move freely.
- Place your arms on the floor by your sides.

3. Loosen the Hinges

"Your spine should move when you breathe, and your pelvis is your energy pump. Your energy cannot circulate with a locked pelvis."[3] Spoken by psychologist and healer Dr. Mitchell May, these words shocked me when I first heard them, after fifteen years of living with a painful, locked upper back. I thought: Your spine is supposed to move when you breathe? I was dumbfounded. That concept changed everything for me.

- Start by finding your three sets of hinges:
  - o One is the "yes-no hinge" at the back of your neck. To find it, shake your head yes and no.
  - o The second hinge is at the back of your waistband. To find it, arch the small of your back off the floor at your waist, keeping hips and upper back on the floor, then flatten your waist on the floor.
  - o The third set is at the front of each hip joint, where thigh bones and pelvis meet. Find these hip hinges by pressing the fingertips of both hands into your hip joints.

- Test your back hinge a few times (this will also test the others):

  o To test the back hinge, with your palm down, slide one hand under the small of your back. Arch the small of your back, and then flatten it. Feel how it lifts off your hand and then presses against it. You do not have to test your "yes-no joint" at the back of your neck. Just keep it in neutral, and your head will get tugged along by the movement of your spine.

  o Go slowly and feel your tailbone roll up and down the floor as you arch and flatten the back of your waist.

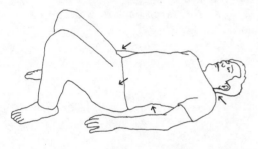

Fig. 11-1. Finding the hinges

Daily Breathing Practice

After you've learned the exercise, do the entire thing with eyes closed, so you can best feel the breath and movement in your body without outside distraction.

STEP ONE: CENTERED BREATH

The purpose of Centered Breath is to establish correct diaphragmatic breathing and coordinate movement of the spine with the breath. The pace is slow and easy. Imagine you are breathing with your whole body and a gentle wave is moving through you.

1. Lie on your back, with knees up and feet flat on the floor, hip-distance apart.

2. Inhale. As you inhale, fill your relaxed abdomen completely as if blowing up a balloon. Round out the space below your waist, between your belly button and the top of your pubic bone.

3. As you inhale, lift your waistline (but not your hips) off the floor, arching the small of your back. Let the movement of your spine follow the breath, rather than breath following the movement of your spine.

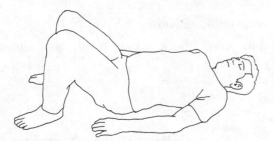

Fig. 11-2a. Inhale, arch back of waist

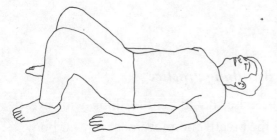

Fig. 11-2b. Exhale, flatten back of waist

4. Exhale. As you exhale, flatten the small of your back against the floor and feel your pelvis tilt up, away from the floor. Do not engage or squeeze your butt, legs, or thighs. This is a breathing exercise, not a butt crunch.

5. Continue inhaling and exhaling slowly, filling your lower abdomen so it rounds out like a balloon while gently arching the small of your back, then exhaling slowly while flattening the small of your back against the floor. The sensations

are subtle, almost like a wave. Let yourself flow into them, feeling your tailbone roll up and down the floor.

6. Practice this for two minutes.

As you begin to make this practice part of your daily routine, you will feel your hinges continue to loosen, as if an old, creaky door hinge has been oiled.

STEP TWO: SPIRAL TWIST

The purpose of the Spiral Twist is to tone and stretch the major joints of the body. Like the Centered Breath, the Spiral Twist is a very slow movement. Imagine a cat stretching and luxuriating, giving herself a bath in a sunlit window.

To learn the exercise, we will do the individual parts of the movement and breathing. At the end, we will put them together into one flowing movement and add breathing.

1. Setup: Lie on your back with knees bent, feet flat on the floor. Put knees and feet together, arms out to your sides in a *T* position, not a *Y*.
2. Arms: Starting and rotating from the shoulders, roll one arm down the floor as the other rolls up. Like two rolling pins, your arms roll in opposite directions, staying on the floor without lifting them.
3. Legs: While keeping your feet on the floor, let your knees drop down on same side as the arm that is rolling down. To remember this, on each side, think to yourself: arm down, knee down.
4. Head: Then add your head and roll it to the opposite side of your dropped-down knees. Rotate, do not lift, your head slowly from one side to the other, keeping it on the floor.
5. Eyes: Move your eyes in the opposite direction of your head.
6. Now put the parts together into one smooth movement.

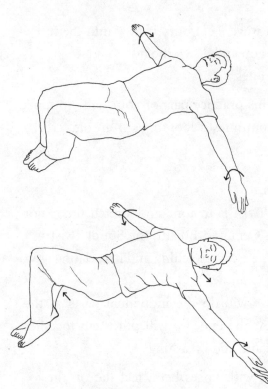

Fig. 11-3a. Spiral Twist, start position

Fig. 11-3b. Spiral Twist, dropped position

7. Breathing: To coordinate the breathing with the movement, do one complete inhale and exhale per side, as knees drop down and come back up.

   • From the center start position: Inhale as knees drop down very slowly to one side, keeping feet in the center. Think: inhale, inhale, inhale.

   • Exhale as you very slowly raise knees back up to the center start position. Think: exhale, exhale, exhale.

   • In order to complete one inhale and one exhale per side, you must slow your pace down by half, then by half again. That should be about right.

8. Spiral Twist: Put everything together and practice for two minutes.

9. Tip: To remember when to inhale and exhale, think about doing resistance exercises or lifting weights when you exhale on the exertion and inhale on the release. In the Spiral Twist, inhale as your knees follow gravity to the floor (release) and exhale as you lift your knees back to center (exertion). In this move, your belly is in its most open, extended position when your knees are dropped to the side, with head and upper body turned in the opposite direction. This allows your belly to round out and expand on the inhale.

STEP THREE: COSMIC JIGGLE

The Cosmic Jiggle increases your circulation and sense of well-being. The pace is quick, like a jiggle. Breathe normally without consciously coordinating your breathing to the movement.

1. Lie on your back, knees up, feet together flat on the floor, arms by your sides.
2. Keep your feet flat and use your heels to push against the floor and generate the jiggle.
3. "Oil" or keep loose your three sets of hinges — your "yes-no joint" or back of your neck, the back of your waist, and your hip joints in front — as you generate movement from your heels toward your head.
4. Jiggle your body in a gentle rocking motion (do not jerk) from head to toe — back and forth, back and forth. Glide horizontally over the floor like a glide-a-rocker.
5. If the hinges are tight, your body will not have much movement, but as they loosen over time, you will jiggle like gelatin.
6. Practice for twenty seconds. It's powerful, so a small amount is enough.

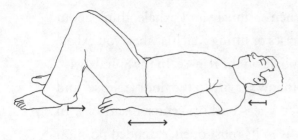

Fig. 11-4. **Cosmic Jiggle**

Step Four: Check-In

The Check-In allows you to notice and feel what the exercise produced for you.

- Lie on your back, legs extended, arms by your sides, and let your body and mind settle.
- Take stock of how you feel. Do you feel different from when you began? What has changed? Are you more relaxed, calm, and peaceful? Do you feel more energized? Are both true? Does your body feel less tense or painful, in general or in a certain area? Do you feel more space in the front of your body, or anywhere else?

Step Five: Sideways Roll-Up

The purpose of the Sideways Roll-Up is to help you transition from lying down to a seated position with a relaxed neck and without contracting the upper body. Use this move to shift from lying down to seated after any activity, such as yoga, breathing, massage, or even sleeping, so you won't tighten everything you just relaxed.

The Sideways Roll-Up is a little like the forward roll-up you do after touching your toes when standing, except you're in a horizontal position on the floor: you roll up one vertebra at a time, starting from the bottom of your spine and moving upward, with your head up last. In the Sideways Roll-Up, you use your arms to push up your torso, while keeping your head and neck tucked until the end, when you're vertical.

1. Lying on your back, bend your knees, feet flat on the floor, and roll over onto your side.
2. Tuck your head and chin to your chest and use your topside arm and hand to begin to push yourself up.
3. When the bottom arm is freed, push yourself up by walking both your hands toward your body, leaving your chin tucked.
4. Let your head and neck unfurl last, when you're finally sitting up.

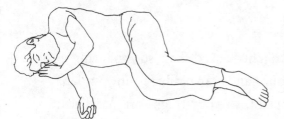

Fig. 11-5a. Sideways Roll-Up, start position

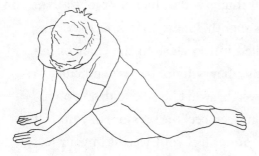

Fig. 11-5b. Sideways Roll-Up, mid position

Breathing in a Chair

Breathing in a Chair adapts Centered Breathing to a vertical position.[4] It promotes relaxed breathing and reduces mind-body stress in your daily seated activities. It counteracts "shoulders to ears" syndrome and head-forward posture — and it's a lifesaver when you're seated at a desk, working at a computer, attending a meeting, or driving.

How to Breathe in a Chair

You will first learn the basic movement and then learn how to make it subtle enough to use while seated anywhere. Begin by putting your body in vertical alignment, so gravity holds your weight. You've already learned how to breathe into your lower abdomen and loosen your hinges in Daily Breathing, so practice that here.

FIND YOUR VERTICAL LINE

In this step you'll situate your chair and your body to support a relaxed, vertical posture.

1. Work with the chair.

    - Sit in an armless, straight-backed chair, so your arms are unrestricted and your hands can easily rest in your lap.

    - Adjust the chair height, so your thighs are parallel to the floor and legs are perpendicular to it. If the chair is too high or low, your thighs will be higher or lower than your knees. (Thighs slightly higher than knees is okay.) If your legs are pulled in too close to the chair or extended too far from it, they will not be perpendicular to the floor, and your weight won't be able to drop down.

    - Always start with your feet. Feel the pressure of your feet on the floor. If you cannot feel your weight in your feet planted solidly on the floor, scoot forward in your chair until you do. Or try adding a folded-up rug, blanket, or firm pillow under your feet if the chair is too tall for you to make good contact with the floor. Feel the pressure of your butt on the seat and your feet on the floor.

    - To support your sacrum, you can insert a small pillow between your lower back and the chair. Keep the pillow *below* your waist. Placing it above your waist and then leaning back against it will produce head-forward posture.

2. Find your vertical line, starting with your feet and seat.

    • Place your feet parallel and hip-distance (at least one foot) apart, with your knees open to create a direct line from your hip joints to your knees, down the legs, and into your ankles and feet. As your weight drops down into your feet instead of remaining high in your shoulders, your pelvis can unlock and gently rock.

    • Sit in neutral on your "sit" bones (ischial tuberosities), the part of the pelvis that your body rests on when you sit. In neutral, the top of your pelvis won't be tipped forward, nor will the bottom of it be rolled in the opposite direction, onto your tailbone. Your weight will be in the middle.

    • Place your ears, shoulders, and hips in a vertical line (as seen from the side). To check for vertical posture, trace a line with your fingers from your ear to the side of your shoulder, then down to the side of your hip bone. Keep your chin in neutral and not tilted up, and slide your head back over your shoulders, so your profile is vertical not diagonal.

ACTIVATE YOUR HINGES

Activate your hinges to allow your spine to move when you breathe.

1. Do you remember your hinges? Two sets, the hip hinge and the back hinge, are involved in Breathing in a Chair because the movement happens from the waist down. To refresh your memory, press your fingers into your hip joints, and then place the back of one hand at the back of your waist. You can also do this with your mind by bringing your attention to them.

2. Now do a seated pelvic tilt: Slowly arch the small of your back as you did on the floor when lifting your waistband.

When seated, basically, you stick out your butt and roll the top of your pelvis forward. Then reverse: roll your tailbone under, letting your low- and mid-back collapse.

3. Repeat.

Breathe into Your Belly

Now put it all together. Breathe into your belly as your spine moves with your breath.

1. Inhale and exhale through your nose, if possible.
2. Breathe into your belly, filling your lower abdomen between your belly button and the top of your pubic bone. (To test for this, place your palm below your waist and feel your belly round out into your hand.)
3. As you inhale, arch the small of your back and tilt your pelvis forward.
4. As you exhale, let your back soften and your pelvis roll under. Let the air escape naturally as if from a balloon; do not push it out.
5. Your movement and range of motion can be big or small, depending on the setting. In other words, no one has to

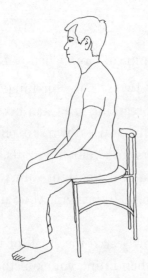

Fig. 11-6a. **Breathing in a Chair, inhale**

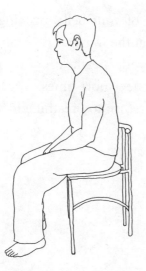

Fig. 11-6b. Breathing in a Chair, exhale

know you are doing it. You will achieve the same results as long as your hinges are activated and your breath is dropped into the lower abdomen.

PRIME THE PUMP (OPTIONAL MOVE)

Use this optional move to get your breath into your belly.

When your belly is not rounding out during the inhale, or you're not sure if it is, you probably are breathing into your chest or very shallowly. If you "prime the pump" once or twice, your breath will just drop into your belly. Use this move whenever your belly is tight and your breath is high (in your chest) and you're not able to shift into belly breathing.

1. Make a fist with your right hand and place it on your stomach *below* your belly button.
2. Place your left hand over your fist.
3. Inhale fully.
4. As you exhale, push your fist into your belly, aiming straight back toward your spine, allowing your breath to make a whooshing sound through your teeth. Using direct pressure,

keep exhaling and pushing air out of your belly, pushing with your fist and bending forward at the waist.

5. Inhale again. What happened? Did your breath "drop" into your belly? Good. Prime the pump a few more times.

6. Once belly breathing is established, return to Breathing in a Chair.

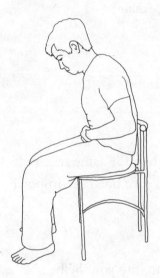

Fig. 11-7. **Priming the Pump**

12 Being Still: Mindfulness and Headaches

Most people have trouble settling their minds, and people with chronic headaches are no exception. The mind just runs along, and when you simply sit quietly, it's like being in a car that has stopped short. All the thoughts, concerns, and emotions you hadn't noticed seem to flood in and hit you all at once. You might feel fearful, anxious, sad, excited, or worried about what has just happened, what might happen, or what is happening now.

What Is Mindfulness Meditation?

Zen master Thích Nhất Hanh describes meditation as the basic practice of "stopping" and finding peace.[1] Stopping helps calm the storm of anxieties, thoughts, and worries that also affect headaches.

Vipassana, from the traditions of Buddhist forest monks in Thailand and Burma, means "clear seeing." This meditation involves clearing the clutter and getting familiar with the mind's landscape. The practitioner focuses attention on the in- and the out-breath, coupled with bringing awareness into the body, as a way to stop, calm, and return to this present moment. Its modern, Western adaptation, called *mindfulness meditation*, is not necessarily part of a religious practice, although its teachings impart the Eastern philosophical principles of equanimity and insight.

Meditation is a way to train your attention, which thus gives you more choice about where you place it. Just like building your biceps at the gym — each time you bring awareness back to your breathing, it's like doing a rep that builds your capacity to focus. If you practice over time, your thoughts and worries will not overtake you quite as easily, nor will they cause such tension in your body.

The Benefits of Meditation

Research studies over the past fifty years have confirmed what ancient Eastern traditions have known for centuries: meditation is good for you. In the 1970s Herbert Benson, MD, found that meditation lowers stress, blood pressure, muscle tension, heart rate, and breathing rate. Recent functional magnetic resonance imaging (fMRI) studies have shown that meditation can alter brain-wave states and pain.

Jon Kabat-Zinn, MD, founder of the Mindfulness-Based Stress Reduction (MBSR) Clinic at the University of Massachusetts Medical School, has pioneered MBSR classes and trainings as part of medical treatment, and his research shows its beneficial effects. Meditation classes are also becoming more widely accepted and available in health and wellness settings for people with cancer, stress and anxiety, chronic pain, addiction, illness, and disease.

Meditating can elicit the kind of relaxation your body and mind crave. You become present, focused, and aware, and you start to notice what is within and around you. You feel rejuvenated and not just running on the proverbial "treadmill of life" in your head. Once you are adept at mindfulness, calming your mind for even five minutes can feel like a mini-vacation.

Cultivating a Practice

Have you ever noticed that you can relax in front of the TV and rest your bones, but not necessarily feel refreshed? Who knew that relaxation was a skill?! Meditation is both the same as and different than simply doing nothing.

Meditation is a skill you master with practice, and, although physically you are "just sitting," it is very different than doing nothing. The difference lies in where you place your attention, and how you use it. Meditation can seem hard, and many people say they are not good at it, but that's because while we're doing it, life comes up. We think about and remember people, places, and things; and we plan. Emotions and memories bubble up. And then we return to the breath. And again and again.

As you practice over time, you *will* get better at noticing what comes up and letting your mind settle into a peaceful state. It's not that your troubles disappear but that your relationship to them and the pull they exert can lift and soften into "being with what is."

As with almost everything, practice makes it easier.

Notice I didn't say, "practice makes perfect"! *Perfection* implies that you are striving to achieve something. In meditation, striving for perfection takes you away from simply being in the moment. Rather than attaining enlightenment or entering into some other state of being, somewhere else, mindfulness is about paying attention in the here and now.

Because thoughts naturally keep arising, sometimes people get discouraged about their inability to meditate, as if it's a talent only some people are born with. They abandon their practice, reporting that they "can't do it very well" and feeling as if they've failed. I often hear this from clients when I begin working with them. This frustrating predicament is actually the best reason to keep going. A practice of returning to the present in your body is a core skill of working with headaches and their associated pain.

The instructions for mindfulness meditation are simple: Pay attention to your body and your breath as you breathe in and as you breathe out — and return your attention to your breath if your mind wanders. And yet mindfulness is more than sitting on a cushion and following the breath. It is a practice of being awake to life in each moment.

Mindfulness Meditation Setup

This section will help you prepare a place to sit that supports your posture in keeping a straight back and staying alert. Read through the entire section before you begin.

Seating

- You can sit on a meditation cushion or in a chair, whichever you find most comfortable. This might vary, depending on whether you are at home, in an office, riding on a train, traveling, or in other settings.

  o With knee or other issues, sitting on a cushion or the floor can be difficult. It's fine to use a chair if you prefer.

  o If you cannot sit, you can lie on your back, arms by your sides, palms facing up.

- In a chair: Have your feet flat on the floor, hip-distance apart, toes facing forward. Scoot forward in the chair, with your thighs parallel and your legs perpendicular to the floor, so your feet make solid contact with it.

- On a cushion: Sit with your legs crossed or in half-lotus or full-lotus position. In half-lotus, one foot is placed on the

opposite thigh; in full-lotus, both feet are placed on opposite thighs.

o   A *zafu*, or firm, kapok-filled meditation cushion, provides a supportive way to sit on the floor because it raises
your seat and hips higher than your legs and keeps your
back straight, posture aligned, and mind alert. (Some
people do cross-legged postures in a chair or on a firm
couch. Here too, use a cushion to raise your hips.)

o   To cushion your knees and feet, you can place the zafu
on a *zabuton*, a flat, rectangular pad, or just use a folded-
up blanket.

•   Align your ears, shoulders, and hips vertically. Proper alignment helps you settle into gravity, reduces upper body
tension, and promotes breathing and alertness.

•   Feel your seat on the chair or cushion, settle in, and let gravity
hold your weight, rather than pulling up and away from it.

Hand Positioning

Position your hands in one of two ways:

•   Fold your hands together in your lap by placing one over the
other and interlacing your thumbs (but don't interlace your
fingers). It doesn't matter which hand is on top; whatever
feels best.

•   Or, place your hands palms up on your thighs. (I advise
against a palms-down position because people tend to grip.)

You Can Use Props

"You can use props, you know," my meditation teacher assured me.
What a relief.

There is no reason to be uncomfortable or suffer pain during meditation. For instance, if your knee sticks up and your thigh and hip joint need support when you're sitting cross-legged on a cushion, wedge a small pillow underneath your knee and/or thigh, so they can rest comfortably. If your arms feel "too short," place a pillow in your lap, whether you're using a chair or a cushion, to support your hands and arms and reduce shoulder strain. When seated in a chair, you can place a small pillow or rolled-up blanket below your waist to support your back if needed. Sitting under your own power instead of leaning against the chair will strengthen your back and core muscles over time.

Every body is different. What is comfortable for you might not be comfortable for someone else, and even what's comfortable for you can vary over time, especially if you have a physical challenge or an injury, or are recovering from an injury. Make modifications as necessary whenever your body needs support.

Mindfulness Meditation Instructions

Now that your body is in position, you're ready to begin. Read through these instructions first, and before you start, set a timer for twenty minutes, so you don't have to keep checking the clock.

- First take three full, relaxing breaths and release each with an "ah" sound. Notice where and how you breathe (chest, stomach, or both? shallow or deep?), and pay attention to the quality and mood of your "ah" (loud or soft? relieved or tired?).
- Now rest your tongue on the roof of your mouth and let your teeth slightly part to soften your jaw.
- Close your eyes and focus your attention on your breath as you inhale and exhale naturally.
  - Breathe through your nose, if possible, to warm and filter the air and not parse the breath.

- o Focus your attention on the filling and emptying of your lower abdomen, below your belly button. Breathe as if a balloon is gently inflating and deflating with each breath.
- o Let your breathing be easy and circular, without any holding between the inhale or exhale.

- When your mind wanders, bring it back to your breath. (It may have been drawn away by a thought, a pain, a noise, or something else.)

- o You might notice your attention wandering within the first seconds of practice, or just a minute before it ends.
- o Whenever you notice your mind wandering, no matter when or how many times during your practice, return your focus to your breathing.

- To complete your practice after the timer goes off, let your eyes come open slowly and let the world come to you.
- Check in with yourself to see what is different. How do you feel, compared to when you started? What do you notice? If you feel calmer and less tense in body and mind, note your feelings and sensations. If you were in pain when you began, has the pain shifted?
- Meditate for twenty minutes, five days per week if possible.

You now know how to meditate, a practice that can set the tone for your day and help you find calm in the midst of chaos and decompress when it is over. You can practice anytime, anywhere, by simply remembering to stop, breathe, and pay attention. Remember to add the time and duration of your practice to your Headache Diary.

Advanced Instructions

Although meditation instructions seem simple, stilling the chatter of the mind is a lifelong practice. My own practice revealed to me how my embodied history could surface as painful sensations that weren't fixed but rather could shift in the moment and over time.

I began vipassana during a particularly challenging time in my life, when I was plumbing the depths of my emotional history as part of my training to become a somatic practitioner. As I got into the practice, I began to feel a burning sensation in my left shoulder during each meditation. When I attended to the burning, I noticed its long oval shape; its location, traversing the "ski slope" between my neck and shoulder; and its shallow depth. I became aware that the burning was preceded by emotionally charged thoughts and feelings of anger about unresolved issues with my mother, which seemed to emerge as my mind quieted.

I followed the instructions for working with pain by focusing on the area and noticing my thoughts without trying to change them. I would feel my pain and stress grow stronger and then move to a different area, and so I would follow it with my attention. Eventually the sensations would dissipate, my thoughts would become calm, and I would return my focus to my breathing. In conjunction, I worked with a therapist and a somatic coach to process my emotions, and as my issues resolved, the burning sensations ceased.

The following two sets of instructions are designed to help you work with pain and discomfort that arise during practice, whether physical or emotional.

Naming

I like making lists. I feel a sense of relief when I write something down (and even more when I've crossed it off), which moves it out of my thoughts and solidifies it in writing, where I can work with it. That is probably why I like the meditation practice of *naming*, also called *labeling* and *noting*. When my mind wanders away from my breathing, naming seems to put a bow on the thought, ties it up neatly, and brings me back to what I was doing: meditating. It breaks the cycle of that thought.

When you find your mind wandering during mindfulness meditation, you can name what it is doing in three ways: *thinking, remembering*, or *planning* — a general way of classifying the type of thoughts you were having based on time. Were you *thinking* about something in the present, *remembering* something from the past, or *planning* for something in the future? Label, name, or note to yourself — "thinking," "remembering," or "planning" — then return to following your breath.

Special Instructions for Working with Pain and Other Sensations

In daily life, we might try to ignore, numb, or retreat from the feelings or sensations that make us feel uncomfortable. As in the story of my burning shoulder, meditation gives us an opportunity to work *with* our pain and discomfort by moving our attention toward it.

When you notice pain or other sensations, bring your attention there, and try to describe what you feel. Keep staying with your sensations and see what happens. Do they get stronger or weaker? Do they change in shape or size? Do they reveal other sensations or emotions as you pay attention? Keep focused on whatever emerges and happens as a result. When the sensations subside or no longer grab your attention, return to following your breathing.

Here's how:

- When sensations arise, focus on them.
- Name the sensations. For example, pain, tingling, itching, pulsation, burning, numbness, stabbing, hot, cold, heavy, light.
- Describe the sensations in the following ways:

- o   size and shape (length, width, depth; on the surface or deep inside; structure; anything else)
- o   intensity (more or less, stronger or weaker)
- o   qualities (for example: feels like a brick, a cord, a sheet-metal plate, a piece of plywood, a bubble; is steady or pulsing, hard or soft, hot or cold)
- o   location (stationary or mobile; stuck, travels, or moves from one side to another)

- Keep following your sensations until they dissipate. Do other sensations, like pain or discomfort, come to the fore? If so, then work with them.
- Do memories, thoughts, or emotions emerge? If so, is there a connection?
- After what you are working with subsides, return to following your breathing.

It is fascinating to discover by direct experience that your pain is not necessarily fixed. It can move and morph when you focus your curiosity and attention on it.

Don't Beat Yourself Up for Falling Off the Cushion

Even when we're seriously committing to a practice — like meditation, a diet, or an exercise program — we can lose focus. Maybe we skip days because we get sick or busy, or we eat something we know we shouldn't. We feel guilty about it and fall off the wagon. Then we mentally beat ourselves up for lapsing: "I'm just not good at this," "My mind wanders too much," "I shouldn't have eaten that; I failed again," "I'll just start again next week."

Don't beat yourself up for falling off the cushion! When you beat yourself up, it just adds another layer of pressure and stress. If you refrain from being so hard on yourself, which can be a practice in itself, you will have more success in climbing back on the cushion. Reframed in the positive: open your heart to yourself. In a 2016 talk on meditation, vipassana teacher Sylvia Boorstein wisely remarked that "the whole of life is a venue for practice" — and, indeed, that view is at the heart of healing headaches.[2]

The Value of Set and Setting

Find a place to do your practices where you can feel at peace and make a boundary if needed. You can create a special space — a dedicated room, a corner of a room, a shelf or altar with meaningful items, a spot in your garden, a bench in a peaceful setting. No matter the size, a quiet, uncluttered sanctuary can free your mind from ordinary space and time.

With busy schedules, work, family, and modern-world demands, a meditation practice is like exercising: if you want it to happen you will likely have to plan it into your schedule. Find a time that works: if you have kids it might be when they are napping or at school, after they are in bed, or when another adult is at home. Share that you are taking some quiet meditation time and close the door.

Maybe your kids, spouse, or partner would like to join you in your practice, if it wouldn't be too disruptive for you. It can be a special time to share together. When children learn to spend five to ten minutes of quiet time in meditation, the calming influence can remain with them throughout their lives.

All that said, you can meditate anytime, anywhere. Sometimes the only choice is to practice on a bus, train, or subway. As you turn inward, the surrounding noises recede. No one has to know. You can wear your shades (or not), close your eyes, and follow your breathing. Just be aware of your surroundings, and don't miss your stop! By the time you reach your destination, you will feel calmer.

13 Posture, Ergonomics, and Sleep

*A*re your daily routines contributing to your headaches and pain? Whether it's sitting for hours at a computer or commuting to work, the way many people use their bodies almost forces them into bad posture. Think of dental assistants and dentists, who bend forward and lean in, unsupported, to work on their patients' teeth. I can imagine their pain.

If you feel sore and stiff at the end of the day or wake up that way, your physical environment and how you position yourself in it could be the problem. Ergonomics is the design of your work environment to fit your body, avoid injury, and promote productivity. Although you might not have the luxury of buying every ergonomically correct product, postural awareness principles will help you improvise and make wise purchasing decisions. If you don't make your surroundings fit you, instead of vice versa, your body will pay the price.

This chapter prompts you to evaluate your daily routines to see if they contribute to your headaches and pain. It covers solutions for many of the physical headache triggers introduced in chapter 7. As you work through these solutions, be aware that when you're beginning to practice aligned posture — whether it's in meditation, breathing, or daily activities — it might feel unnatural. This seems to be a common phenomenon, and it makes sense. You have practiced your uniquely misaligned posture forever and your body is used to it, so anything different, even supportive posture, can feel odd until you log enough time to reap the benefits of bodily ease. You are changing the relationship of your body in space and gravity, and it's finding a new equilibrium.

When you make postural or ergonomic changes, note them in your diary, along with any results.

Perils of the *C*-Curve

We perform most tasks with our arms out in front while facing what we're doing, whether that's driving, typing, texting, writing, reading, cleaning, cooking, feeding a baby, or playing an instrument. That's good. The problem is, as we do them, we're often out of alignment, leaning in toward the activity. This creates the *C*-curve.

Viewed in profile, this misaligned torso is "*C*-shaped" in both length and width, with head, neck, shoulders, and arms pulled forward, chest and ribs collapsed, mid-back rounded, and tailbone tucked under. Over time, this head-forward posture produces pain, fatigue, numbness, and muscle imbalance. It's like holding a bowling ball out in front of your body and carrying it around. The muscles and fascia in the shoulders, neck, and lower skull are constantly contracted and get built up, just like biceps curls build arms — but in this case, they get built because you're out of alignment! This buildup can become so dense that the head is unable to pull back over the shoulders and begins to form a premature hump over the C6 and C7 vertebrae.

Whether you're leaning forward or back, if your head and neck are held in front of your body, the *C*-curve happens. When you lean back in an executive chair or a driver's seat, ostensibly to relax, your head also has to come forward in order to see what you're doing. The head-forward posture can also result from what we carry. Children begin carrying backpacks early, starting with five pounds of books and supplies in grade school and continuing through high school and college, where they might lug around eighteen to thirty pounds. In order to avoid being pulled over backward by the weight, they lean over at the waist with the upper body pulled forward for balance. And finally, lest we forget, we're often in bent-neck posture while texting, using smartphones, and viewing other electronic devices. This is creating postural problems for all ages, but these days it's starting younger.

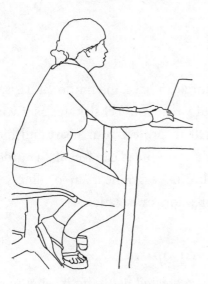

Fig. 13-1. Seated, legs tucked, leaning forward, arms extended

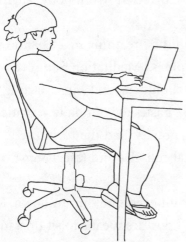

Fig. 13-2. Seated, leaning back, head and arms extended

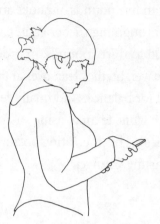

Fig. 13-3. **Texting with bent neck**

In other cases, *C*-curve posture can have an emotional basis; it can be tied to mood or take hold when you feel sick. It's as if your upper body is curling in on itself to protect your heart and hide your vulnerability. Even holding up your head can feel like a burden if you have been dealing with chronic migraine, pain, or illness or have feelings of resignation, depression, or isolation.

Align Your Spine

Fortunately, a *C*-curve can be corrected with body alignment practices.

You learned postural basics in the Breathing in a Chair exercise (on page 153) and in the Mindfulness Meditation Setup (on page 162): vertically align your head, shoulders, and hips, starting with your feet. You can also apply these basics to your daily activities. An aligned spine allows your bones, gravity, and the furniture to support and hold your weight so that muscles and fascia aren't forced to do more than their share.

Whether seated or standing, not everyone slumps down. Many of us are taught that having good posture means to sit or stand up as straight as possible. But this postural habit of stretching up and away from the pull of gravity makes your muscles and fascia work harder than necessary. Regularly practicing meditation, Breathing in a Chair, and healthy ergonomics will increase your comfort with using gravity to settle your weight while aligned, instead of trying to pull up and out of it.

But how can you maintain your alignment once you find it? Your posture changes with your activities, and you can't just find an ideal position and maintain it all day without moving! You're not a statue, and a held stance is as harmful as a misaligned one. If you are working on your computer, don't you eventually end up leaning into the screen, even when you're trying to stay aligned? We all lose track of our bodies when we're absorbed in what we're doing.

The solution is to make an attention loop, whereby you monitor your posture and make little shifts instead of trying to hold your alignment static. Periodically shift your attention from your current activity and bring your awareness back into your body to see how and where it is positioned. If needed, make corrections to realign, and then return your attention back to your activity. It's not a one-off. Keep coming back to your body throughout your day; it only takes a second. I am always having to bring my head back over my shoulders and pull my eyes away from the computer screen. Like all the practices you are learning, the more you tune in to your body and shift it, the less you will have to *think* about doing it, and the sooner it will become second nature.

Using Postural Principles in Daily Life

Now that you know the basics, you can adapt them to any activity, from working to relaxing. Again, every body is different.

If you keep postural principles in mind when you buy or use items in your daily life, you can make choices that support *your* body in alignment. When you purchase an item that entails sitting, such as a car, couch, or chair, choose one that fits your body. To make your current items fit better, try to adjust or modify them. The way you carry your stuff and how much you carry matters. Be mindful of what you carry, from heavy purses to backpacks and briefcases, lest you risk undoing your other good habits. If you wake up with headaches or migraines, evaluate your sleeping posture and bedding as potential triggers as well.

Even what you wear can modify how your body fits in its surroundings. Various shoe heights (flats, heels, platforms, boots, or sneakers) and clothing thicknesses (a bulky coat versus a thin summer dress) will affect where and how your body sits relative to the floor and your seating. To compensate, adjust your surroundings to fit your body: car seat, distance from the gas pedal, steering wheel tilt; couch and chair pillow support; desk seating and keyboard height.

Now let's look at how to apply postural principles to some common situations.

Sitting at Your Desk

Problems arise when you start modifying your posture to fit surroundings that are ergonomically incorrect for you, producing bodily strain and tension. So often, people put up with something they know is wrong because they feel powerless to change it. But there is often something you can do. Whether your workplace is inside or outside your home, do whatever you can to adjust your workspace to suit your body.

Always begin with the basics, as in Breathing in a Chair (page 153): Vertically align your head over your shoulders and stack your torso, letting your weight drop down into your seat and feet. Let your chin drop and lengthen, meaning extend, the back of your neck.

Relax your upper arms against the sides of your torso, with your lower arms parallel to the floor and resting on your lap or keyboard. If you are short-statured, try a keyboard pullout tray. When your keyboard is situated too high, you raise your arms and shoulders, creating tension there and in your neck. Don't use office chair arm-rests, for the same reason.

When typing, place your wrists at the same height as your hands or slightly higher, or use a wrist rest. Contracting the back of your wrists and positioning them lower than your hands can cause irri-tation, pain, and repetitive strain injury.

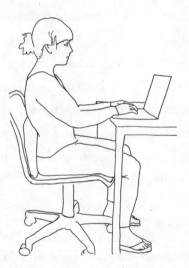

Fig. 13-4. **Seated at computer, aligned posture**

Incorrect desk and monitor height can hurt you. Sometimes you have to make give-and-take adjustments between the heights of your chair, desk, and monitor, depending on what you are work-ing with. Position your screen at eye level, where you can look at it without having to tilt your chin up, which contracts your neck and shoulders. If your monitor is on a stand or riser that forces you to constantly look up, change your setup. View your screen looking straight ahead or aiming your gaze slightly downward; this is often easier on a laptop, as long as you don't hunch over.

Face your work. If you have worked with the same setup for years without giving it a second thought and you end up sore after a day's work, now's the time to reevaluate it. Do not let your environment dictate the position of your body. Make it work for you. If your equipment and supplies (monitor, phone, paperwork, stapler) are set off to the side and you regularly twist your head to work with them while your torso, arms, and hands are doing their work straight ahead, your body is in a torqued position. As a result, you are contracting and straining muscles and fascia in your upper back, arms, shoulders, neck, and lower skull. We can get so used to this kind of habitual movement (often made under a time crunch) that we don't recognize its perilous effects.

One way to solve the torqued-body problem is to use a tool I learned about in massage school: your "belly button flashlight." Imagine you have a flashlight in your belly button. Always point your flashlight at your hands to illuminate them — and face your head in the same direction. It will keep you from getting twisted out of shape when doing just about anything.

Relaxing

Sometimes we put our bodies in positions that hurt us even when we think we are relaxing! For instance, a teenage client of mine had the habit of using her laptop while lying in bed on her stomach with the back of her neck and shoulders scrunched up as she looked at the screen. She had no idea that her habit was contributing to her headaches.

How do you use your body when you relax? Do you lie down on one side while propping up your head with your bent arm to read?

That crooks your neck. Is your couch or easy chair so soft that you sink down into it? That's a C-curve in the making.

When you're relaxing on a couch, lying in bed, watching television, reading a book, playing computer games, using your smartphone, cruising around in your car, or riding your bike, use the postural principles you have learned — props, pillows, and all.

From Cars to Couches: Considering Posture in Your Purchases

If you are eyeing a major purchase, such as a car, couch, easy chair, mattress, or other furniture, do your research first, and fit the item to your body. Also consider your body in the decisions you make when you are renting a car, traveling, or sleeping away from home.

When I was car shopping, I noticed that the cars from a particular company were designed with the driver's seat upright position tilted back at a thirty-degree angle. Knowing that leaning back in the seat would force my head forward while driving, I did not choose that brand. Some cars did not have a height adjustment feature to raise the driver's seat, which forced me to extend my neck to see above the wheel. And seating with built-in support did not always suit my body. Good ergonomics was a key factor in making my choice.

The softest couch is not necessarily the best for relaxing. When couch shopping, I found myself sinking down into some styles, while others were too deep for my height. I felt like a little kid in giant furniture, knees above my hips, feet suspended off the floor, with insufficient back support. I knew that if I purchased one of these styles, my body would suffer, so after "kissing a lot of frogs" I finally found a comfy couch and pillows that supported my alignment.

Whether it's a car or a couch, find what works for you, keeping in mind that your body's needs can change.

What You Carry

A heavy purse, briefcase, or backpack carried over one shoulder can throw off your posture and pull your body down on one side. Then in order to stand straight, you have to contract your muscles to hold your shoulder up with an amount of force against gravity that matches the weight of the bag pulling it down; otherwise the bag would slide off. Or you adopt a misaligned posture, with one shoulder dropped as you carry the bag. A cross-body bag is good, but if it's too heavy, the strap will pull on your neck and shoulders, which will contract to counteract the weight.

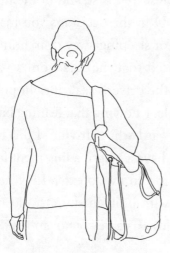

Fig. 13-5. Backpack side-carry, misaligned posture

Do you really need everything in your bag? Before leaving your home, office, or car, always ask yourself: How much do I really need for this particular trip? If you're just going from the car into the restaurant, for example, can you remove some of the things in your bag and leave them in the car? Eliminate anything you will not be using. Do you really need to carry that giant purse to do errands or go to an appointment? Can you carry a smaller bag and leave the tote in your car or office? Can you better distribute the weight with two smaller bags? Some handbags are heavy even when they are empty. It all adds up. Carry a lighter bag, wallet, and key fob; use travel-size lotions; and take fewer makeup items.

If possible, opt to roll your luggage, computer, paperwork, and supplies instead of hauling them through the airport or other destination. No doubt, some schoolkids won't think it's cool, but a rolling backpack to transport their heavy schoolbooks is far easier on their shoulders, back, and posture — and thus their headaches. Perhaps e-readers can replace some or all of the heavy schoolbooks that they carry.

How Do You Sleep?

If you wake up with headaches or migraines or have disrupted sleep, your sleeping posture could be contributing. To avoid shoulder, neck, jaw, and lower skull tension during sleep, you need a supportive bed and pillow. Of course, the experience and perception of what is supportive is different for everyone, and so are each person's requirements for sound sleeping.

Here are some general guidelines to follow when choosing your bed and pillow or determining if they are triggers. First, when you lie down, your neck, head, and spine should be in a straight line, just as when you are upright.

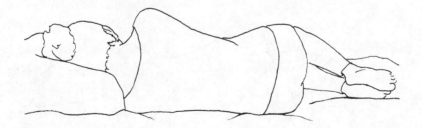

Fig. 13-6. Lying down, aligned spine

If your mattress is too soft, your hips and shoulders will sink down into it, causing your spine to bow. If it is too hard, your hips and shoulders will be pushed up, unable to sink down into the mattress, which will curve your spine the other way. Both positions keep your spine out of alignment, putting strain and tension in your neck, shoulders, and back whenever you sleep or lie down. Your mattress should allow your shoulders and hips to be supported and yet sink in enough to keep your spine straight.

Pillow height is a big deal — and it's all relative to your body. If your pillow is too soft, low, or thin (for you), the top of your head will tilt down. If your pillow is too tall, thick, or hard (for you), your head will tilt up. Either way, this misalignment pulls and contracts muscles and fascia in the sides of your neck and top of your shoulders.

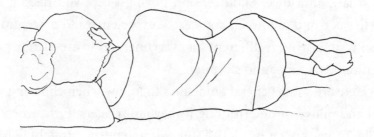

Fig. 13-7a. Lying down, pillow too high

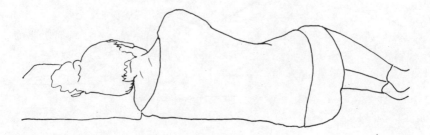

Fig. 13-7b. Lying down, pillow too low

When lying on your side, make sure your pillow lies at the height needed to support the sides of your neck and keep your head in line with your spine. Your head should sink down into the pillow so your head lies flat and your neck is straight. Cervical pillows are designed for that function and are shaped to take up the space between the neck and bed to keep the cervical spine straight. Like everything, including bodies, pillows are made in a variety of shapes and sizes, so no single one will uniformly fit everyone. Try them out in the store to find what is right for you.

14 The Zen of Exercise and Headaches

*E*xercise — or lack of it — is a common headache trigger. This chapter provides loosening exercises you can do sitting or standing, and exercise support strategies to get you moving again.

People who have had headaches for many years, especially migraine, might have cut back on exercising because they haven't felt up to it. However, lack of exercise contributes to bodily tension and weakness, poor mood and outlook, stress buildup, and sluggishness. Even light movement does the opposite; it increases circulation, aids digestion, brightens mood, reduces stress, and boosts energy levels.

Stephen Gaskin, who cofounded The Farm, used to say, "Pay attention to the square-inch field." That's a helpful way to frame your thinking when starting to exercise following periods of inactivity due to pain, illness, or injury. First handle what is closest to you — the "square-inch field" around yourself. Make that good, then extend yourself out from there. Gaskin's advice for people who want to save the world is to start right where you are: when you get up in the morning, first make your bed, brush your teeth, and then see what else needs to be done. You don't need to conquer everything at once, just put one foot in front of the other.

Applying this advice to exercise: start small and pay attention to your body. When you can handle a short period of mild activity, without negative side effects, you can take on a bit more. Whenever you step it up a bit, stay at that level for a while, so your body can integrate it.

This way of handling life by living in the moment, being aware of everything around you yet still being attuned within yourself, is akin to Zen Buddhism. When you're present you can make adjustments accordingly. It's about being aware of your body's messages and subtleties, rather than determinedly pushing through. You feel your edge and go with the flow instead of forcing it.

Track what you do. Remember to add what, when, and how long you do any exercise into your Headache Diary — as well as any aftereffects: tired, energized, loose, tight, sore (and where), satisfied.

Loosen-Up Exercises

The following sets of exercises will loosen your shoulders, neck, head, and face, ease habitual holding patterns, and increase mobility and flexibility. You can do the whole set or mix and match. If you have a tension headache or feel one coming on, select several that would feel good and do those. *Note:* If a migraine is impending or you are in the midst of one, do not do these now; wait until you feel better.

Incorporate these exercises into your daily headache prevention routine, and also use them on the go to loosen up tight spots. You can rotate them, doing different exercises on different days, or you can do a partial set mid-morning while taking a five-minute break at your desk, then do another few in the afternoon or at lunch. Once you start doing them, you will likely discover stuck, held, contracted, and painful areas or points that you were unaware of before. By creating more movement and flow, you will run more energy through your body, increase your circulation and flexibility, and decrease your chances of injury, pain, and fatigue. Don't worry about what you look like doing them; just have fun. Children will love them too!

Face Play

If you have a job where you always have to be "on" with a helpful face and a smile, or if you habitually hide your true feelings or discomfort in real-life situations, you could be wearing a virtual mask. Over time it becomes a habit: you forget that your face was holding a tense position, and it still is. I call it "social face." Face Play melts away the mask, and it also relieves facial and eye tension caused by intensive computer work or driving.

Tune in to your body as you do these exercises. Breathe naturally, and if you notice you're not breathing, start! If any exercise seems difficult to do, it could be because your face is tight. Try to let go in those areas, and just go for it. *Note:* If you have TMD/TMJ, pace yourself. Start slowly, don't push your jaws to the edge of their range, and pay attention to how your joint responds.

How to Do Face Play

- Blow through your lips. Make a sound like a horse. Then blow through your lips while humming. Feel your lips and cheeks vibrate.
- Soften your mouth and lips and make a humming, vibrating sound through them while rapidly vibrating or shaking your head "no."
- Play with your mouth, and tongue in and out while making sounds. Feel the vibrations in your mouth, throat, and chin area.
- Make a pop-cork sound by pulling your index finger outwardly from your slightly tightened opposite cheek. Repeat five times on each side.

- Raise both eyebrows and your forehead and then let them down. Repeat ten times.
- Squeeze your eyes shut and keep them closed while scrunching up your nose and mouth, then open your eyes and relax your face. Repeat five times.
- Open your eyes wide, hold, then relax and close them. Repeat five times.
- Lion's pose with face: Look straight ahead. Open your mouth and eyes wide, stick out your tongue toward your chin, raise your brows and forehead, and look up. Hold. Repeat three times.
- Flutter your eyelids rapidly, keeping eyes, eye area, and face soft without squeezing for about five seconds.
- Follow your finger: Do two to four passes of each of the following moves while keeping your head in the middle.

  o Straighten your index finger, hold it about six to eight inches from your face, and follow your fingertip with your eyes, tracing a line slowly in the following directions: up and down, side to side, diagonally from top right to bottom left and back, diagonally from top left to bottom right and back, and figure eights, starting from between your eyes outward, first in one direction, then in the opposite direction.
  o End the exercises by closing your eyes softly and breathing; then open them slowly.

Desk Exercises

You are probably familiar with many of the following exercises as warm-ups, but they are also great to use at your desk as stand-alone exercises, or as a way to just get up and move when you are working, studying, or traveling.[1] Do the whole routine daily as a preventative.

Or if you feel tight or stuck, do a set of shoulder or head rolls on the spot. Mix it up, keep it fun, get loose!

You can sit or stand for seven of these, and four are done while standing. Do an equal number of repetitions per side. The recommended numbers are listed, but listen to your body to determine what is right for you.

Take it slow and easy. Relax your body; stack your head, shoulders, and hips; soften your knees; and remember to breathe. Look straight ahead and let your chin drop instead of tilting it up. Do not push to the edge of your range if a movement makes you tighter. Instead, reduce your range of motion by making the movement smaller — and go more slowly. If any exercise produces pain, discontinue it.

To Do Seated or Standing

- Shoulder raise, single: Raise your right shoulder all the way up as you inhale, then let it drop as you exhale. Repeat five to ten times and switch sides.
- Shoulder raise, double: Raise both shoulders as you inhale, then let them drop as you exhale. Repeat five to ten times.
- Shoulder roll, single: Roll right shoulder backward five to ten times as you breathe slowly, then forward five to ten times. Repeat on the left side.
- Shoulder roll, double: Roll both shoulders backward five to ten times, breathing slowly. Repeat, rolling forward.
- Head tilt: Look straight ahead and bring your ears in line with your shoulders, keeping your chin down, not lifted. Very slowly tilt your right ear toward your right shoulder as you inhale, then return your head to the middle as you exhale. Repeat five times, then switch sides.
- Head roll, lower half circle: Do this exercise very slowly, in a half circle (not a full one).

- o Starting with your head in the center position, drop your chin toward your chest, then inhale as you roll your head toward your right shoulder, raising your head to the top of its range above your shoulder, as your chin tilts up.
- o Exhale as you let your head roll down again slowly to the middle starting position.
- o Repeat the instructions as you continue the roll very slowly on the left side.
- o Repeat three or four times, ending with your head in the center down position. (Do not do an upper half-circle roll.)
- Yes-no joint: Activate the "yes-no joint" in your neck. Slowly shake your head "yes" five times, gently moving it up and down, then "no" five times, gently moving it side to side. Repeat once or twice. You can even say the words *yes* and *no* to the movement. It's freeing and might make you smile!

To Do While Standing

- Swimming: Plant your feet hip-distance apart, with knees bent, shoulders relaxed, and arms by your sides. Moving from your shoulders, use your arms to swim the crawl stroke: right, then left, one stroke after the other. Repeat ten times.
- Cat stretch: With your feet hip-distance apart and your knees bent, bend over at the waist, placing your palms on or above your knees. Slowly arch your back as you inhale, stretch the front of your neck upward, and hold. Then round your back out as you exhale, drawing in your belly, and hold. Repeat five to ten times.
  - o Roll-up: From the rounded cat-stretch position, beginning at your hips, slowly roll back up vertebra by vertebra, unfurling your low, mid, and upper back, neck, and,

lastly, your head. Inhale and exhale as you readjust to standing up.

- Look far: Place your feet about six inches apart, with your knees soft, body stacked, shoulders relaxed, breath dropped, arms by your sides, and head level. Look straight ahead.

  o Very slowly begin to turn your head to the right without lifting your chin. Let your eyes start and lead the movement, with your shoulders and then your torso following along, twisting toward the back as if wringing out a towel. Breathe naturally and keep your shoulders down and open.

  o When you have reached your limit, remain in that position, still looking far to the back as you relax and breathe.

  o Take three deep breaths, and, again leading with your eyes, slowly return your head and body to center, and take two or three more breaths.

  o Repeat to the left.

Isometrics

Isometrics are resistance exercises that counterbalance muscle contraction with equal force — so there is a stretch but with no movement. You simply contract then relax your muscles, which produces an effect similar to that of progressive muscle relaxation. The sets below help release muscles that extend through your neck and attach to your lower skull, shoulders, and chest.

Sit in a chair or stand with your body vertically aligned. Remember to breathe, and don't tense your face or the rest of your body during isometrics.

HEAD PRESS: FRONT POSITION

Place one hand over the other and rest them, palms down, across your forehead, elbows out to the side. Push your head straight forward as if it's a glide-a-rocker, making sure your chin is not tilted up. At the same time, push toward the back with your hands and arms, exerting equal force. Your head will be static and won't move. Continuing with your breathing, hold for a count of ten seconds, and then release.

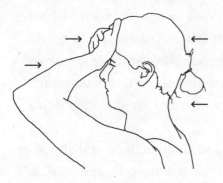

Fig. 14-1. **Isometric front head press**

HEAD PRESS: BACK POSITION

Place your hands, one palm over the other or fingers laced, on the flat area at the back of your head. Holding your elbows out to the side, simultaneously push your head straight back, making sure your chin is not pointed up, and push forward with your hands using equal force. Your head will be static and won't move. Continuing with your breathing, hold for a count of ten seconds, and then release.

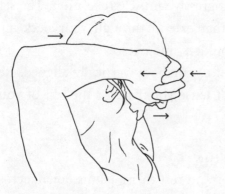

Fig. 14-2. **Isometric back head press**

HEAD PRESS: SIDE POSITION

Do the head press on the side of your head, each side separately. (First re-stack your body, so your ears, shoulders, and hips are vertically aligned.) On the right side, flatten your right palm and place it above your right ear, elbow held diagonally. Push your head to the right against your hand while pushing your hand against your head, using equal pressure. Your head will remain level and in the middle. Hold for a count of ten seconds, breathing naturally, then release. Repeat on the left side.

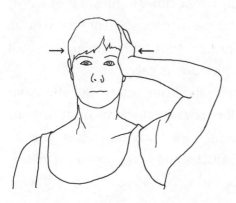

Fig. 14-3. Isometric side head press

Just a Walk around the Block

To break a cycle of inactivity, begin slowly and do not push it. Remember the square-inch field? Start small. Just take a walk around the block; the change of scenery can work wonders. In addition to building strength and stamina, walking releases feel-good hormones that can instantly improve mood and make you feel more in control of your headaches and pain. Of course, listening to music or having a congenial walking partner helps pass the time and gets you out of your head. The key is to listen to your body before you begin and throughout your walk (or whatever exercise you choose).

Try this strategy: Decide you're going to take a walk just to the end of the block. When you get there, see how you feel. If you feel okay, round the corner and walk one more block. If you feel like continuing, walk around one square block while listening to your body's signals. If you feel better by the time you reach each corner, keep going. If you feel your energy start to wane, turn around and go back home (unless you're almost there)...or take a rest.

Remember, however far you get away from your starting point, you are only halfway to the finish line, so be sure to reserve enough energy for the return. As you get stronger, increase your routine from ten minutes out and ten minutes back, to fifteen, twenty, and thirty minutes each way. I set my phone timer to ring at the halfway point of the total amount of time I want to walk. Do not try to break any speed or time records — just get your body moving gently. If you are doing okay, feel free to pick up the pace.

Stretch your legs, back, torso, and arms before and after your workout. Gentle stretching before a workout warms up your body and promotes mobility in your muscles, fascia, and joints. Stretching afterward lengthens your muscles and keeps you from getting stiff.

Pace Yourself

When some headache patients, especially migraineurs, start feeling better, they tend to get so enthused about finally being unburdened from their pain that they exercise longer and more vigorously than they are used to. They often lose themselves in activities and forget to drink water or eat — or they do more than their bodies can tolerate, which makes them tighten up afterward. Doing too much, too soon can be a trap because they end up having a setback. To best help headaches, it's good to loosen up and get moving gently and incrementally.

If you push yourself too quickly, you might end up taking one step forward and two steps back. Remember, slow and steady wins the race. If you do a little at a time, you won't get ahead of yourself, use up your reserves, or suffer the consequences of your body tightening up. Pace yourself and keep noticing how you feel before, during, and after you exercise.

Enjoy Yourself!

Think outside the box exercise-wise. Find an activity you like, in a place you enjoy. For instance, you can take a walk by the river, along the shore at the beach, in a park, or around your neighborhood. If you enjoy a gym workout or class, go there. In addition to standard fare, many gyms offer a variety of classes, such as yoga, Pilates, tai chi, and dance. If you don't belong to a gym or it's not your cup of tea, find a dance studio, movement center, or Meetup group that offers what you like.

If you're not sure what you like or where to go, do some research. Many centers and studios offer discounts or free classes or events that you can try before you buy. Each teacher, center, and studio is unique. If you want a certain style of dance, movement, or yoga, for example, but you don't groove with a particular teacher or studio, don't give up; keep searching until you find one that is right for you.

An exercise buddy or group can also be a motivator to get you out and moving, make your routine more enjoyable, and help the time pass quickly. Try to find someone who walks or works out at a similar pace, so you don't push yourself, lose track of how you're feeling, and overdo it. Enjoy the freedom of being able to move without pain, and keep moving in order to prevent it.

Part Four

Hands On:
The Healing Power
of Touch

15 Touch Prep: Listening with Your Hands

*I*n these next five chapters, I convey my hands-on headache heal-ing wisdom and heretofore esoteric techniques for pain relief and prevention, using precise steps accompanied by illustrations, diagrams, and annotations.

Everything you have learned so far is part of your tool kit: you know how to shift into wonder mode, be your own headache detec-tive, eat a headache-healthy diet, breathe, meditate, align your pos-ture, and gently exercise. Not only will these practices prevent your cycles of pain and help you feel more calm, confident, and relaxed, but they will also support and ground you in learning how to work with your touch.

This chapter shows how to use your pain as a signpost and your mindful touch as the vehicle to reach it. If that left shoulder keeps burning, you can apply touch instead of reaching for medication. You can explore the qualities of the pain: What, where, when, and how is it? Is it hot, cold, or numb? Does it feel like a hard knot, a piece of two-by-four lumber, or a sheet-metal plate?

Working with Your Pain

Most people have no idea how much tension they regularly hold in their shoulders, neck, head, and face, nor do they understand the connection between their tension and their headaches and migraines. They might finally become aware of it at the point of feeling pain, or they might stay tight and held in one position for so long that they even become numb to the pain. Our fight-or-flight response reads the pain as a danger signal, so it's combated with medication or ignored. In light of all that, the idea of working *with* pain might seem backward.

Touch is a language all its own. Like a forgotten art, the power of touch to relieve aches, pains, and bodily tension is underrated, undervalued, and underused. As a result, we are out of touch with ourselves, literally and figuratively — so much so that we forget to try it or doubt that it could even be effective. This makes sense because we are not taught how to use touch or receive it. Just as a pianist could not play a concert at Carnegie Hall without years of practice, no one can master the subtleties of touch just from reading a book. But one can begin.

Although it might sound counterintuitive, you can use touch and awareness to locate and move *toward* instead of *away from* your pain in order to relieve it. That is why breathing and meditation are so foundational to touch therapy; they build your capacity to focus on your body and your pain — and now, your touch.

In addition to using the terms *massage* and *self-massage*, I often describe what we're doing here as *touch, touch therapy, mindful touch, bodywork, somatic bodywork*, and *hands-on work*. These therapeutic modalities encompass and combine techniques, such as energy work, breathing, awareness, deep-tissue massage, holds and pressures, myofascial release therapy, movement, and dialogue. They reflect a participatory and interactive framework of using bodywork for transformation on many levels.

Mindful touch is different than zoning out or falling asleep to relax. It has special powers. When you bring your attention into your pain as you work on it, your touch's ability to affect it becomes amplified. And when you feel your pain easing under your touch, you will know what is effective and be able to replicate it. I always combine touch and awareness, no matter what modality or who I'm working on.

The body has four types of tissue: connective, muscle, nervous, and epithelial. When you apply touch you are making contact with them all, which is why I often refer to *tissue* instead of *muscle* in bodywork. One kind of connective tissue, called *fascia*, is especially important in pain relief and prevention, as you will see later in this chapter.

Touch Prep

In touch therapy, as with most things, it's not what you do but how you do it that matters. Touch Prep is a series of techniques that helps you sensitize your hands and attune your focus, so you can effectively bring touch and awareness right to your pain and relieve it using the instructions in chapters 16 through 19.

You will be working with sensations and qualities of tissue that can be *felt* on the body and the head. Rather than solely using terms from anatomy and massage, I describe these subtle experiences and techniques with familiar terms and playful names, accompanied by a few anatomical references. We'll start with "Puppy Dog Paws" and "Little Frog Pads," two foundational Mundo touch techniques that are key to any great massage. They're easy and fun to remember.

Puppy Dog Paws

Puppy Dog Paws are soft, pliable hands. Just imagine the paws of a begging puppy.

Like creates like. Soft hands help you blend with the tissue, listen for what's tight, and release it. Tight hands cannot soften bodily tension because they can't blend with, listen for, or ease out what is tight. As a result, they force the tissue, which can produce more tension, residual soreness, and pain — just the opposite of what you want.

How to Make Puppy Dog Paws

Hold your upper arms against the sides of your torso, bend your forearms up at the elbows, and flop your hands palms down, mimicking a begging puppy. (I even make a whimpering sound!)

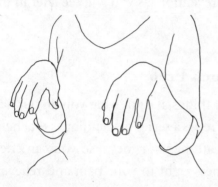

Fig. 15-1. **Puppy Dog Paws**

Soft Hands Test

To make sure your hands are soft, do this test:

1. Turn your palms down and place your right palm over the back of your left hand.
2. Brush your left hand out and upward from under your right palm. If both hands are soft, your right hand will flop back down like a puppy dog paw.
3. Reverse hands, placing your left palm over the back of your right hand. In an outward, upward motion, brush your right hand out from under your left palm. Your left hand should flop back down.
4. Repeat a few times back and forth, then return to making Puppy Dog Paws.

CLAW HANDS TEST

Now test for tight hands, the kind you *don't* want to have.

1. Place your left hand on your thigh.
2. Make your right hand into a claw and latch it onto the back of your left hand.
3. Make little circles with your right hand. Feel how the fingers of your claw hand poke into the back of your left hand? Your right hand has limited sensitivity and contact, can't get in deeply, and covers a limited area.
4. Return both hands to Puppy Dog Paws.

Little Frog Pads

Little Frog Pads is a technique that helps you latch onto the skin in order to go more deeply into tight, painful points and areas. The name comes from little tree frogs native to Puerto Rico (coqui) that live in rain forests. They have tiny toes that act like those rubber darts with suction cups, so they will stick to wet leaves and not slide off.

HOW TO MAKE LITTLE FROG PADS

1. First, make Puppy Dog Paws.
2. Then place your left hand on your thigh, palm down.
3. Place the finger pads, not the tips, of your right hand on the back of your left hand, in the webbed skin between the bones.
4. Latch onto the surface of your skin, making good contact.
5. While latched on, make little circles and back-and-forth moves in the webbed areas. Use your skin as a point of contact to get in more deeply to the underlying layers of tissue. Latching on is different than *effleurage*, the gliding, circular,

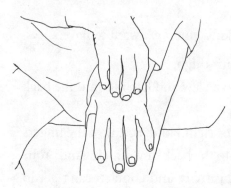

Fig. 15-2. Little Frog Pads

light-touch massage stroke used to apply lotion to the skin. Pretend that you are applying lotion to the back of your hand. Although this is soothing, notice that your touch is more on the surface and does not go in deeply, as with Little Frog Pads. Then resume Little Frog Pads and feel the difference.

When you squeeze an avocado or a peach to see if it's ripe, you are not testing the skin but merely using the skin as a point of contact to test the flesh inside. You are listening with touch to assess what is beneath the skin and how much it gives, which is exactly what Puppy Dog Paws and Little Frog Pads allow you to do: you latch onto and blend with the surface of the skin in order to work with the tissue beneath it.

You don't have to do the Puppy Dog Paws, Soft Hands Test, Claw Hands Test, or Little Frog Pads exercises each time. Use them at first and anytime you are not sure whether your hands are soft, tight, or latched on. During self-massage and hands-on headache therapy, keep monitoring your hands and soften them if you tighten up.

Energize Your Hands

This simple technique wakes up your touch by warming your hands. Energize your hands each time you do bodywork until you are able to warm them with your mind.

How to Energize Your Hands

1. Make Puppy Dog Paws, then press your palms together firmly.
2. Focus on your palms, keep pressing, and rub them together briskly until heated.
3. Then place your hands on your thighs, palms up.
4. Bring your awareness into both palms. What sensations do you feel? Heat? Tingling? Pressure?
5. If you don't feel anything, repeat the process until sensations come into your palms.

With practice you will be able to energize and warm your hands by simply bringing your attention into your palms, without rubbing them together.

Listen with Your Hands

Yes, you can listen with your hands — and actually use them like ears! You will get lots of information if you simply pay attention to your hands and get curious about what they are contacting.

How to Listen with Your Hands

- Clear your mind and "listen" with your hands to the quality of tissue you are touching. Notice what it feels like — hard, soft, tight, loose.
  - o For example, reach across in front and squeeze the ridge of your opposite shoulder between your fingers and the heel of your palm.
  - o Is it soft on the surface but hard a few layers in, or is your shoulder rock-solid throughout? Do you notice other qualities or anything else?
- If you find a tight spot, notice its size and shape. Notice where it is, whether it's near the surface or deeper in. (You learned

this focusing technique as part of the advanced instructions for meditation in chapter 12, in the section "Special Instructions for Working with Pain and Other Sensations" on page 167. Now you are simply adding your touch to it.)

- When you work on a painful spot, does it soften, dissipate, move, or reveal another painful spot?

The information you get from your body by listening with your hands will guide you in deciding whether to stay on the same spot or move to another.

The Three Bears of Touch

The Three Bears of Touch is an analogy to help you gauge how much pressure to use. In the story of Goldilocks and the Three Bears, one bed was too hard, one was too soft, and one was just right. The amount of pressure used in touch can be described in that way too.

- *Too hard:* When you use too much pressure or work too fast, your body resists. If you suffer through a painful massage, thinking that deeper is better, but then end up sore afterward, that is also too hard. A "more pain, more gain" philosophy is counterproductive because your body tightens up in protection to avoid being hurt.
- *Too soft:* If the pressure is too light, it is ineffective and can feel annoying and uncomfortable, which in itself produces stress.
- *Just right:* Just right is using only the amount of pressure it takes to contact your tightness or pain without making more. If you are causing more pain than you had to begin with, the pressure is too hard. If you are not making contact with your pain, the pressure is too light. Pressure that is just right lets your body relax enough to let the touch in, and lets you go deeper without producing more pain.

- The right amount of pressure cannot be measured on a scale because each area you work on can require a different amount, and this can change from day to day and moment to moment.

Attention and Communication

Attention and communication take place on many levels in bodywork — between the giver and receiver, between your touch and the tissue you are working on, and in the body's responses to that touch.

In massage, there's a giver (the therapist) and a receiver (the client), but in self-massage you play both roles. To do so, you must split your attention between what you are touching as giver and how you are experiencing that touch as receiver.

Science and psychology define this as *interoception* and *exteroception*. As both the giver and receiver of a self-massage treatment, you have the unique ability to experience the effects of your touch on your body from the inside (interoception) and from the outside (exteroception) at the same time. In self-massage, you are coming from the outside with your touch and matching it up to the pain that you are feeling on the inside. In other words, while you are working on your shoulder, which feels like a rock from the outside and is sore from the inside, you can also feel the *effects* of your work concurrently — on the outside with your touch (the tissue feels softer and warmer) and on the inside with your perception (your tension and pain are relieved). The entire process is you paying attention in each moment as your touch communicates with your body and then paying attention to the changes that result from your touch.

It's delightful that once you learn, you can give yourself exactly what you need, just how you want it.

Touch Biofeedback

In biofeedback, patients learn to reduce their stress and produce mind-body integration by breathing, meditating, and hand warming and can read the results through a computer program, wearable device, or phone app. These biofeedback devices use sensors to measure brain waves, muscle tension, temperature, respiration, and perspiration, giving instant feedback with a tone or readout display.

The process of focusing and bringing your attention and touch to your body is like *touch biofeedback*. In self-massage and hands-on headache therapy, you use your hands and body as biofeedback sensors, from which you get real-time information. By bringing your touch and awareness to your pain and working on it, you produce, as in typical biofeedback, a new result, including changes in breathing, muscle tension, pain, circulation, and the color, tone, and texture of your skin. Your awareness of those changes serves as your readout. Ask yourself: What changed, and where and how is the pain now? The immediate, direct internal and external effects of each therapeutic move will serve as guidance to inform your next one.

You Can't Hurry Fascia

Let's return to the fascinating world of fascia, a kind of connective tissue. Fascia is the spiderweb-like matrix that encases your muscles at every level — cell, bundle, and group — as well as your internal organs, holding them in place throughout your body. If you have ever prepared to cook chicken, you might have noticed the thin, strong, gelatinous tissue attached to the flesh, almost like plastic wrap — that's fascia.

Made from the same kind of tissue as blood, bone, and cartilage, fascia knits together and responds to stress and relaxation, warmth and cold, thoughts and touch, breathing and awareness, and more. By working with fascia using touch therapy, referred to as *myofascial* (literally, muscle-fascia) therapy, you can ease the tension and tightness that contribute to headaches and migraines.

Did you ever play with Chinese finger traps, those tubular puzzles made of woven straw? You stick an index finger into each end, and when you try to pull your fingers out, the trap constricts and grabs them. The harder you pull, the tighter it grips, and you are stuck until you figure out the puzzle. The trick is to ease both fingers inward, then out very slowly. Working with fascia is similar because you can't rush things, and if you try, it will tighten up.

Working with fascia is also like catching a moving train: you have to match its speed in order to jump on. It's a very slow train, and its speed is relative. The tighter the tissue, the slower it goes. Fascia's lesson is that your body is not in a fixed state; it is always responding, and you can aid it with your touch. Latching onto your skin and experiencing the sensations of your tissue easing, melting, and moving will accelerate your ability to relieve your pain in the moment and prevent it in the future.

The Secret of Painless Deep Massage

The next two techniques, Ease into the Tissue and Find the Floor and Work There, are my secret sauce for painless deep massage. They provide a gentle way to release deep layers of tightness, holding, and tension without any aftereffects of lingering pain.

These techniques build on The Three Bears of Touch because they help you determine how much pressure is "just right" for each painful or tight spot, so you can reach the heart of it without resistance. That's because when you're using these techniques, your body does not tighten up to protect itself from the discomfort of too much pressure or working too deeply, too fast. (If you notice your hands tightening up when applying any technique, remember to soften them into Puppy Dog Paws.)

Ease into the Tissue

Easing into the Tissue relies on sensitivity and communication, not power or strength. Therefore, always invite the tissue to respond; never force your way in. To do this, move very slowly into ever-deepening layers of tissue, using only the amount of pressure it takes to make contact with your pain and tightness without making more. If you create more pain than you had, lighten up on the pressure and slow down your movement.

Find the Floor and Work There

When you start working on your pain, you might be surprised to discover that a seemingly singular painful area, your shoulder ridge for example, is actually made up of a collection of painful points. To release the whole area, you have to release each point within it. Use Find the Floor and Work There to alleviate the pain in each point when you follow the self-massage instructions in chapter 16.

Here's how:

1. Ease into the tissue by applying pressure just to the depth at which you meet resistance or pain, called *the floor*.
2. Apply steady pressure, Little Circles, or Back-and-Forths, according to the massage instructions, at the floor, or point of resistance, without pressing harder or making more pain.
3. Continue working at that depth of pressure until the tissue warms, softens, and becomes more pliable, and your pain eases.
4. Then apply a bit more pressure and go deeper.
5. Find the new floor, the new point of resistance, and determine if the point is still painful or has released. If it's still painful or tight, then work at *that* depth of pressure. Never force your way in. Only go in as deeply as the tissue will allow.

6. Keep repeating the process of finding the floor and easing that point until the pain, soreness, and tension are gone. When that point feels warm, soft, malleable, and pain-free instead of tender, tight, and painful, you have reached the ground floor.

7. To exit that point, release the pressure gradually and with ease.

8. Locate the next point that feels painful to you and repeat this process or complete the massage.

Each area you work on can have a different sensitivity. Some areas (and some people) are more sensitive and need a slower, lighter touch than others. For example, the sides of your neck are more delicate than your shoulders, but even so, some people's tight shoulders can tolerate only extremely light touch. For many migraineurs, too much pressure or a too-deep massage can even provoke a migraine afterward — which is another reason to use these techniques.

Shake It Out!

Self-healers must empty their hands and arms of what they collect while working on their bodies.

At the end of and during your hands-on session, it's natural for your hands and arms to get tired. After all, you've used them to collect all that pain, tightness, tension, fatigue, and stuck energy from your body. In order to release it, you have to dump it out, like the trash. This technique shows how to get rid of it.

How to Shake It Out!

Always get rid of what you collect by shaking out your hands and arms in this special way when they get tired. Shake out each arm separately.

1. Bend your forearm up at the elbow, so your hand is held softly in front of your shoulder.
2. Straighten your arm swiftly with a spiral motion and extend it to the side and diagonally downward toward the floor, palm down, fingers and thumb fully extended.
3. Shake your arm like you mean it! Flick your hand like you're trying to get rid of something stuck to your fingers. Accentuate the movement on the "out, out, out" to forcefully direct what you've collected out through your arm, hand, and the tips of your outstretched fingers.
4. Treat what you get rid of like real stuff, and don't shake it onto yourself or anyone else. Shake it toward a window, body of water, corner of a room, or floor-wall intersection. (Give yourself plenty of room, so you don't whack yourself on the furniture.)

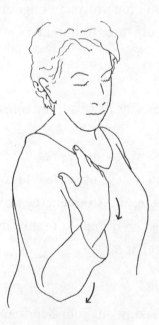

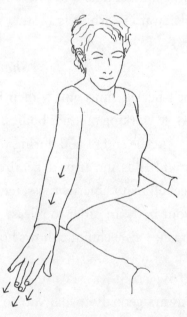

Fig. 15-3a. Shake It Out!, start position

Fig. 15-3b. Shake It Out!, end position

5. Keep repeating this move until your arms feel refreshed and are no longer tired or sore.

6. Then resume or complete your self-massage or headache therapy.

It's surprising how much "stuff" you can collect! You will know how much there is by how tired your arms and hands feel. It can take several repetitions on each side to empty them out.

Exploratory Mode

Earlier in this chapter, I discussed how working on and with your own pain is challenging and exciting because you are both the giver and receiver of treatment.

Exploratory Mode returns us to beginner's mind — this time applying it to the realm of touch. In order to effectively quell your own pain, you must step out of its grip, get curious about its qualities, and work with it as a sensation or set of sensations. By exploring pain as sensation — how deep, wide, hard, or soft is it? what shape is it? — you can actually feel a real-time shift and change your pain.

Is your pain stuck, or does it move? Does a memory, a thought, or an emotion surface as you work on a troublesome spot? As you reenter beginner's mind and get curious about the what, where, when, why, and how of your body and your pain, keep listening to and exploring what emerges.

Approach

The way you approach your body and your pain matters — and so do you. *You* matter. Approach your body with care. You are not just working on a collection of parts; you are entering into a life-energy field, and your body reflects your history and your experience. Your hands receive information and are effective not only when your touch is relaxed and energized, but when your mood is calm and your mind is open.

How to Approach Your Body

- *Be fully present.* Information about how and where to touch unfolds through a neutral channel that is open to receiving information. To open that channel, quiet your thinking mind. As in meditation, put your mind into neutral and don't question yourself. If you're thinking or worrying, even about whether you are doing it right, you're one step removed from being present to your touch and its effects.
- *Work from general to specific.* Think of working on your body like working with clay; clay is difficult to knead when cold but malleable and easy to shape when warm. Your body is the same way. Begin by warming and softening an entire area, using the process to assess individual hot spots. After the area is warmed and loosened, work specifically on the tight, tender, painful spots you've identified.
- *Create a loop of awareness.* Notice what your hands are feeling under their touch, how your body feels and responds to the work — and what your hands feel as your body changes. Also keep coming back to your standard practices: align your posture, breathe into your belly, let gravity hold your weight, soften your hands. Then refocus your awareness on where your hands are working.

16 Relieving and Preventing Pain with Upper Body Self-Massage

*I*n chapter 15, you learned the foundational skills needed to master the intriguing touch therapies you will use for headache relief and prevention. This chapter covers self-massage techniques, routines, and application instructions for the shoulders, upper back, upper arms, chest, and neck.

After covering which technique to use when, I will teach you a variety of massage strokes, holds, squeezes, and pressures — based in deep-tissue, myofascial, and energy-work techniques — which we'll then combine into therapeutic routines. Working from general to specific, the techniques are used to warm, soften, and assess the tissue, and to move more deeply into hot spots to release them.

Even if only one side of your head or body bothers you, always work on both sides to release buildup and create balance. You might be surprised at what you discover. For instance, the shoulder that doesn't hurt as much can get tight from overuse because you're trying to avoid using the shoulder that hurts. So work on them both.

The techniques in this chapter (and in chapter 17) work best with short nails, at about one-sixteenth of an inch, so you don't poke yourself. (Even one-eighth of an inch can be a bit long.)

Benefits and Usage

In addition to relieving upper body tension, stiffness, and spasms that often contribute to headaches, massage therapy provides a cornucopia of benefits in headache relief and overall health: it increases circulation; enhances immune system functioning; improves mood and mental alertness; lowers blood pressure, tension, and stress; releases habitual postural and internal holding patterns; and increases mind-body awareness and sense of well-being.

How to Use Self-Massage

Use the self-massage techniques and routines in this chapter (16) and the next (17) to:

- Relieve an active tension headache
- Relieve and prevent neck, shoulder, chest, head, and face tension and pain
- Prevent tension headaches and migraines by eliminating the upper body tightness and holding that contribute to them
- Relieve the tension-headache components of migraine, sometimes referred to as "migraine with neck-related (or *cervicogenic*) symptoms"
- Reverse an emerging tension headache or migraine before it escalates
- Release the stuck pain symptoms of a migraine from the neck and lower skull in preparation for a Mundo Method application on the front of the head

How Not to Use Self-Massage

Do not use self-massage for migraine.

Unless you are releasing the stuck pain from your neck or lower skull to prepare for the Mundo Method, do not use self-massage during a migraine. Self-massage is too intense with too much movement to use on a migraine, which needs a more subtle and quieting technique.

To relieve an active migraine, follow the Mundo Method instructions in chapters 18 and 19.

How Often to Do Self-Massage

At the beginning, practice every day, or at least five days per week.

If your body is tight, sore, or numb most of the time and you have frequent headaches or migraine episodes, try to do some self-massage every day. You can do the whole routine in one sitting, or do parts of it throughout the day. You can target different areas on different days — for example: neck, or neck and shoulders, on one day, head massage on another; face massage on one day, and chest and upper back on another.

As you incorporate all the stress-reduction practices into your routine, you can begin to rotate between meditation, breathing, and self-massage. It's all maintenance. As your body loosens and your headaches and pain subside, you can cut back on the self-massage frequency. If you notice tightness building up again, then increase your sessions accordingly.

Self-Massage Instructions
The Basics

Always begin with the basics. Sitting in a supportive position immediately addresses the bodily stress and strain, muscular contraction, and fascial tightness that build up from head-forward posture and chest breathing. If you keep returning to stacked posture during self-massage, you will save yourself a lot of work, as well as muscular buildup and tightness in general. So return to the following as often as you need:

- Center yourself vertically in a chair, starting with your feet. (See page 154.)
- Soften the area around your jaw by resting your tongue on the roof of your mouth, with your teeth slightly parted.
- Breathe into your belly, and let go of all thoughts. (See chapter 11, page 156.)
- Make Puppy Dog Paws and energize your hands to wake them up. (See page 201.)

Shoulders

- The shoulder girdle is made up of the area between your clavicle (collarbone) in front and scapula (shoulder blade, sometimes called the angel's wing) in back.
- Work on each shoulder, using the opposite side hand and arm so you will not engage the muscles on the side you are trying to relax.
    - Reach around the front of your body to your opposite shoulder.
    - Relax your arm and elbow, letting the upper arm rest on your chest, so you're not holding it or your shoulder up.

SHOULDER SQUEEZE-AND-HOLD

This generalized hold warms and softens the shoulder ridge and upper arm:

1. Grab a hunk of shoulder ridge (the trapezius muscle) between the heel of your hand and your fingers.
2. Squeeze, using the *flats* of your fingers up through the first knuckle, not your fingertips.

3. Keep squeezing your shoulder ridge and pull it up and away from your body toward the ceiling. (I call it "pulling the meat off the bone.") Feel your shoulder warm and soften inside your grip.

4. Hold each grip for about ten seconds (one one-thousand, two one-thousand...), as you breathe, then release. With each hold, breathe into your belly, inhale and exhale through the nose, or in through the nose and out through the mouth with a sigh, lips soft and not pursed.

5. Relax your working shoulder, arm, and hand.

6. Repeat the Squeeze-and-Hold, this time moving out to the end of your shoulder, then your upper arm (deltoid muscle — where you can use your thumb in front, instead of the heel of your hand), and then back toward your neck. End on the "ski slope," where the top of your shoulder ridge begins to slope up toward the neck.

7. Shake out your working hand and arm when they get tired or filled up — anytime along the way or after completing one side. (See chapter 15, page 211.)

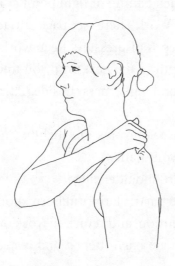

Fig. 16-1. Squeeze-and-Hold and Squeeze-Release along shoulder ridge

SHOULDER SQUEEZE-RELEASE

This is a quick, rhythmic version of Squeeze-and-Hold.

1. Hold for a second, or the time it takes to say "squeeze-release."
2. As you do this, move rhythmically along the ridge.
3. Do Squeeze-Release along your shoulder ridge and down into the upper arm (again using your thumb in front) to further loosen, warm, and break up congestion.
4. You can do Squeeze-and-Hold on both sides, followed by Squeeze-Release on both sides, or do both moves on one side, followed by both moves on the other side.

LITTLE CIRCLES

This circular technique is useful for going deeper into a tight or sore point using Touch Prep in chapter 15 (see page 201). In this case, you're working on your shoulders, but you'll also use it on other areas.

1. Latching on with Little Frog Pads (either under or over your clothing), hold your fingers together as a unit.
2. Staying latched on, move your fingers in little rhythmic circles, circling outward (for shoulders).
3. Using Little Circles, ease into each painful or tight point as it softens. Use Find the Floor and Work There (see page 210) to release the point to the next depth of pressure. Keep working on that point from one depth to the next until you find the bottom floor and the pain and tenderness subside. Then find the next point.
4. To move between points, release your pressure slightly (instead of lifting and re-placing your hands).
5. Do Little Circles along the entire shoulder ridge.
6. Repeat on the other side. Note particularly stubborn spots that might need additional attention, and return to work on them more deeply after the tissue has softened and rested (like clay or bread dough).

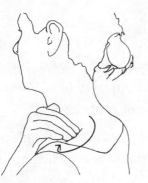

Fig. 16-2. Little Circles along shoulder ridge

BACK-AND-FORTHS

This back-and-forth move loosens congestion and habitual holding; use it as an alternative move to Little Circles.

1. Holding fingers together as one unit, latch onto the skin with Little Frog Pads.
2. Move the tissue back and forth with a gentle, repeating, rhythmic tug-and-release movement.
3. You may find that some areas feel better or are easier to reach with Back-and-Forths; others, with Little Circles. Experiment with both until you find what works. Both of these techniques are good on the shoulders, upper back, back of the neck, and scalp.

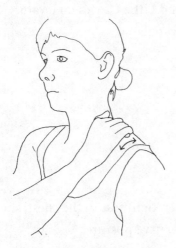

Fig. 16-3. Back-and-Forths on shoulder and upper back, fingers moving vertically

BACK OF THE SHOULDER / UPPER BACK

Repeat the entire shoulder routine, this time on the *back* of the shoulder and along the scapular ridge (the top ledge of the scapula, or shoulder blade). Work with the opposite hand, your arm extended across and resting on the front of your chest.

1. Place the heel of your hand along the front of your shoulder, palm on your shoulder ridge and the flats of your fingers along the back of your shoulder and scapular ridge.

2. Do Squeeze-and-Hold, Squeeze-Release, Little Circles, and Back-and-Forths.

3. Switch sides and repeat.

4. Do Little Circles and Back-and-Forths on the inside top corner of the scapula, a typical hot spot, where the levator scapulae muscle attaches. (The other end is attached to your upper neck, or cervical vertebrae — C1, C2, and C3).

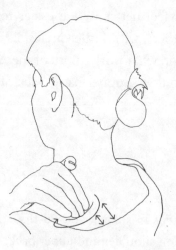

Fig. 16-4. Back-and-Forths and Little Circles on levator scapula.

Chest

The following moves release and open tightness in the chest, shoulders, and upper back and address *C*-curve posture.

Upper Chest Taps

This technique breaks up tissue congestion and holding and enlivens and brings more energy into your chest area.

1. With your upper arm by your side, bend your elbow and turn the palm toward your chest. Fingers are relaxed and slightly curved, turned vertically, and separated about a quarter-inch.

2. Tap lightly across your collarbone (clavicle) and upper chest to gently release it and the heart area. Tap lightly like a pediatrician taps on the chest when listening to a child's lungs with a stethoscope. Let the vibrations of the taps go inward.

3. Tap up and down the breastbone (sternum).

4. Emphasize the contact part of the tapping motion, to go *in, in, in*.

5. Feel the tapping vibrate inside, enliven your chest area, and expand your breathing.

6. This movement covers the entire chest, but you can repeat it with your other hand.

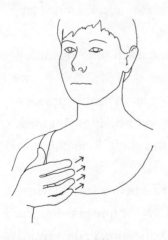

Fig. 16-5a. Upper Chest Taps, hand lifted in preparation

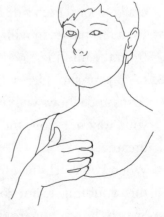

Fig. 16-5b. Upper Chest Taps, hand tapping on chest

Sternum and Clavicle Stretch

This technique releases tight fascia, addresses head-forward posture and C-curve, and opens the chest and heart area. It is done on both sides at the same time.

1. Curving your fingers (make Puppy Dog Paws) and separating them a quarter inch, position your hands in the middle of your chest on the breastbone; your fingers will be placed vertically, facing back-to-back.

2. Check your posture and alignment, and correct any head-forward position. Align ears, shoulders, and hips.

3. Elbows are by your sides, shoulders down and relaxed.

4. Press in with all fingers, latching onto the skin (or on top of your clothing), and make contact with the underlying tissue. Keep pressing in steadily but gently while exerting outward traction to stretch and ease out the fascia. Go only as fast as the tissue lets you; feel the melt.

5. To move laterally to the next area, release pressure slightly while still holding outward traction.

6. Repeating this press-stretch-and-release motion, move laterally toward each side of your chest.

7. Do a few passes moving up your chest, each time beginning from the midline.

8. Keep your shoulders relaxed and your arms near your sides. Arms and elbows will rise away from your body as you work your way out from the middle of the chest. Remember to breathe.

9. When you reach the top couple of ribs below your clavicle, turn your fingers horizontally to follow the line of your ribs.

10. Switch the traction from an outward direction to downward diagonally as you press and release your fingers; then work your way up over the clavicle in the same way.

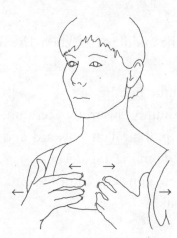

Fig. 16-6. Sternum Stretch, horizontal traction

11. Keep starting with both hands at the middle, each working its way outward to the edges of your chest as you exert downward traction.
12. You can work your way down again if desired.
13. Feel your chest open and your head settle back over your shoulders.

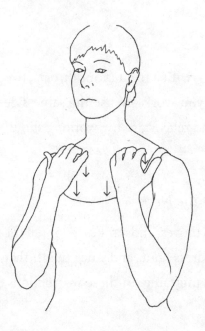

Fig. 16-7. Clavicle Pull-Down, vertical traction

Spider Silk Pull

This technique expands and opens the middle of the chest. Use your dominant hand.

1. To activate the area, tap the sternum lightly.
2. Next, curve hand, fingers, and thumb toward the sternum, then bring them together and pull straight outward and away from you, as if grasping and pulling a spider silk.
3. Let the middle of your chest follow along and come forward, as if being tugged along by the silk.

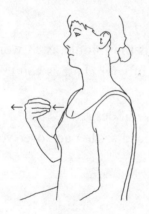

Fig. 16-8. Spider Silk Pull, **away from chest**

Neck

Work on your neck as if it's a box — with a front (your throat), two sides, and a back. Whichever side you work on, use the same-side arm. Keep both shoulders down and relaxed, so the working shoulder is not raised.

The Back of the Neck

Apply this series of holds, squeezes, moves, and strokes to loosen the neck and the lower skull, and to address knots and stuck points that herald tension-type headache and migraine. In these instructions, we begin on the right side.

KITTY-SCRUFF HOLD

This version of Squeeze-and-Hold warms and softens tissue at the back of the neck. In Kitty-Scruff Hold, you hold yourself by the scruff of the neck, like a kitty, but instead of pulling up toward the ceiling as in Shoulder Squeeze-and-Hold, you squeeze and pull back and away from the neck as if toward a wall.

1. Curve your right hand and fingers into a *U* or hook shape, and mold them to the back of your neck. Your wrist and the heel of your hand will be against the back of your right ear, and your bent arm will be on the diagonal, held away from your face.

2. Grab and squeeze the back of your neck between the heel of your hand on the right side and the flats of your fingers on the left. Your thumb isn't part of this grip; instead it rests alongside your hand.

3. Continue to squeeze, pulling straight back and holding your grip like a mama cat carrying her kitten.

4. Breathe and keep holding as you feel the tissue soften and warm.

5. When the tissue eases, release your grip and repeat this hold along the length of your neck, working up to the bottom of your skull and down to the base of the back of your neck.

6. Use your thumb and fingers to continue over the protruding C6 and C7 vertebrae, in a pinching, squeezing motion to break up tissue congestion.

7. Switch hands and repeat on the other side.

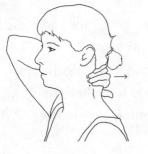

Fig. 16-9. Kitty-Scruff Hold and Squeeze-Release, pulling away from neck

SQUEEZE-RELEASE

Next, apply Squeeze-Release (see page 220) to the back of your neck to warm, soften, and loosen it.

1. Use the same arm and hooked-hand position as in Kitty-Scruff Hold.
2. Do Squeeze-Release rhythmically up and down the back of the neck. You can do several passes.
3. Switch hands and repeat on the other side.

THREE STRIPS UP THE BACK OF THE NECK

This move uses Little Circles and Back-and-Forths to get deeper into tender, sore, painful points and find hot spots to return to for deeper, more specific work. Starting at the top of the neck, you'll work on the three strips following a down-up-down direction.

1. Use the same arm and hooked-hand position as Kitty-Scruff Hold. Stack your fingers vertically and use them together as one unit.
2. Think of the back of your neck as the back of a box, divided in the middle by your spine. You will massage three "strips" on each side of it.
3. To find the middle, trace along your spine with your right-hand fingers from the protruding C6 and C7 bones up to where your spine meets the bottom of your skull.
4. Then slide your fingers out slightly to the right of your spine and find the valley that runs just next to it.
5. Using three fingers, latch on with Little Frog Pads and press in to make contact with any tightness or pain.
6. Do Little Circles in an outward direction, releasing the pressure slightly as your fingers spiral down to the next spot. Keep repeating until you reach the bottom of your neck.

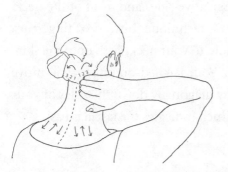

Fig. 16-10. **Three Strips Up the Back of the Neck (down, up, down)**

7. Do Little Circles on top of and around C6 and C7 to loosen congestion and buildup.
8. For the second strip, slide fingers to the right of C7 from the first strip over to the middle of the right side of the box.
9. Again latch on and do Little Circles, spiraling back up to the bottom of the skull.
10. For the third strip, slide fingers outward to what would be the right edge of the box. Latch on and do Little Circles down to where the neck and shoulder meet.
11. Repeat Three Strips on the left side using your left hand.
12. After completing one side or both sides, return to any remaining tender or sore points and work on them using Little Circles and Find the Floor and Work There (chapter 15, see page 210).

The Sides of the Neck

People tend to think their "pain in the neck" emanates from the back — until they start working on the sides. You might be surprised to find that tight fascia surrounding the protruding muscle that runs diagonally from behind your ear to the top of your chest, called your sternocleidomastoid, or SCM, is often responsible for your neck pain.

To handle the more delicate, sensitive sides and front of the neck, I use a special Gentle Glide-Release technique. Instead of fingertips, use the "flats" of your fingers to mold to your neck, latch onto the skin, and release the tissue underneath. Your latched-on fingers will move extremely slowly, inching their way diagonally down the sides of your neck, powered solely by gravity, which indicates the fascia is easing.

Gentle Glide-Release

Use this flat-finger, super-slow technique to release pain and tightness and increase mobility.

To locate your SCM for the first time, start up-top behind your ears, near the bottom of your protruding mastoid bone on either side. Make a channel between the side of your bent index finger and the pad of your thumb, place this channel at the bottom of the mastoid, and *gently* pinch and release. You'll feel the top of the SCM there; keep lightly pinching and releasing along its length diagonally down both sides of your neck, where it ends at the collarbone. Now you know where the SCM is.

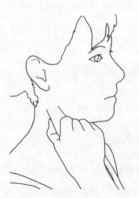

Fig. 16-11. **Channel Stroke to find the SCM**

How to Do Gentle Glide-Release

1. Do both sides at once to provide balance, so your neck muscles don't engage.
2. With your fingertips together as one unit, position them on the SCM at the bottom of the mastoid bone, behind each

ear. Mold the flats of your fingers along your SCM, keeping hands and fingers soft, so they drape your neck.

3. Press in and latch onto your skin, using it to make contact with the fascia underneath.

4. Relax your shoulders, with upper arms resting on your chest. The weight of your arms being pulled down by gravity provides gentle traction as your latched-on fingers follow the SCM's diagonal line *without* gliding over the surface.

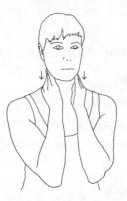

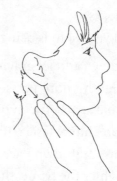

Fig. 16-12a. Gentle Glide-Release start position

Fig. 16-12b. Gentle Glide-Release of upper SCM

5. The trick is to achieve a balance between downward traction and pressing in with the flats of your fingers. When you find that midpoint between pressure and traction, the tissue begins to release *inside* and your fingers will move. To your touch, the Glide-Release can feel like the tissue is easing, oozing, stretching, and melting. When you get it just right, your fingers will move at glacier speed down the sides of your neck.

6. When the flats of your fingers reach one-third of the way down the SCM, reposition your fingertips there, remolding them and your hands to your neck, and continue the technique.

7. At two-thirds of the way down, reposition your fingers again and continue the technique until you reach the collarbone.

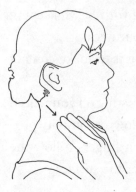

Fig. 16-12c. Gentle Glide-Release, reposition at one-third and then two-thirds of the way down the SCM

FINE POINTS

If you feel your skin is being pulled or stretched instead of melting:

- Slow down and let gravity do the work.
- Try slightly more pressure while slowing down to find an equal balance between pressing in and downward traction.
- You can't hurry fascia. It hates deadlines. You just have to let it release at its own pace.
- The tighter the tissue, the slower it goes.

BERMUDA TRIANGLE

This technique releases the scalene muscles and fascia in the oft-forgotten triangular-shaped area behind the SCM and in front of the trapezius muscle, which slopes between the neck and shoulder. Continuing the neck-as-box analogy, this area would be at the back of the sides of the box. I call it The Bermuda Triangle.

1. Using both hands, place your fingers on the sides of your neck at the bottom of your skull, in the valley behind your SCM.
2. Apply Gentle Glide-Release in a forward direction horizontally. Remember to move at glacier speed and keep breathing.
3. When you reach the SCM, reposition your fingers an inch lower at the back corner of the sides of the box, and apply Gentle-Glide Release horizontally on that swath.

4. Keep moving down until you've covered the whole triangle between the trapezius and the SCM.

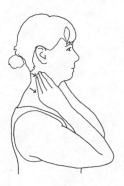

Fig. 16-13. Gentle Glide-Release of Bermuda Triangle, behind the SCM

How Do You Feel?

Taking a few moments for self-assessment, ask yourself: "How do I feel now? Compared to when I started this massage, what feels different?" By taking stock of how you feel and what has shifted, you will reap more benefit from the treatment. Feeling the results breeds hope for a pain-free future and will build confidence in your ability to create it.

After you take stock, record in your diary the time (and date) of your session, what you did and for how long, and of course the results. For example: "left shoulder looser, softer" (or "sore") or "neck still tight, tired" or "relaxed, energized." Note any changes that occur over time.

I developed many of these routines, methods, and techniques by working on myself, lying down, for as long as it took to get relief. In some cases, that was hours at a time. If your body is particularly tight, sore, and painful, working on yourself in lying-down position is an effective way to release it. It puts your body in a horizontal neutral position, where you're probably more used to relaxing.

Sometimes, you just have to put in the time. Your body will reward you.

17   Relax Your Head and Face

*I*n this chapter the head and face get special attention. The fifth
and largest cranial nerve, called the trigeminal nerve, is located
in the forehead, temples, eye area, and upper and lower jaws. It
partly controls chewing and biting functions and the sensations
in the face. This three-branched nerve and its related blood vessels
play a large role in the mechanism of migraine as well as tension
headache.

The techniques for working on the head and face become pro-
gressively more subtle. In addition to head and face massage routines, this chapter will teach you how to complete any self-massage
in the "Massage Closing and Assessment" section. The "Next Steps"
section helps you assess whether you have done enough or should
work on the headache itself with the Mundo Method. The chapter ends with short-form instructions for the routines presented in
chapters 16 and 17. You can use these instructions for easy reference
after you've learned the techniques in these chapters.

As with shoulder and neck self-massage, the techniques in this
chapter might be inappropriate for migraine because they involve
too much movement. The only exception would be when you
need to release a stuck migraine from the neck or lower skull. For

guidance on "How to Use Self-Massage," please refer to page 216 at the beginning of chapter 16.

The Head

Heavy thinkers and worriers tend to tighten their scalp, forehead, or both, which can make them more vulnerable to tension headache and migraine. Calming your thoughts and worries with meditation can reduce the amount of tension in your head. Head massage is another way to loosen and ease out taut, tender, sore, or stuck points or areas of your scalp. The object is to get your scalp to move.

The head is delicate, so approach it with care and gentle touch. The occipital, parietal, and temporal bones form the back of your skull, with muscles that attach there and extend into your neck. When you palpate your skull, you will notice anatomical lumps, bumps, and what's commonly known to massage therapists as the occipital ridge, which feels like a ledge right above where your skull slopes down toward your neck. This area contains lots of hot spots because of the muscle attachments and because the fascia tightens in protection when we're stressed.

Setup for Head Massage

- Remove or loosen hair ties and clips to allow for freer scalp movement.
- Imagine the head as a box, with back, sides, and top. Focus on all these surfaces to make sure the entire scalp gets attention.
- Work on both sides simultaneously, using your rounded finger pads and not the tips. Work your fingers in unison, like a tool.
- Latch onto your scalp underneath your hair (not on top of

it) to make good contact and move easily between points or holds.

Methods

- Loosen the scalp by moving it over the surface of the skull.
- Use an even amount of pressure. Working with the scalp is different than going into ever-deepening layers of tissue, as in upper body self-massage.
- Make just enough contact to move your scalp. Don't press so hard as to make extra pain.
- To move your scalp if it's stuck: As with the Gentle Glide stroke in chapter 16, find a balance between how hard you press and, in this case, the circular or back-and-forth movement. In concept it's similar to the Cosmic Jiggle, step 3 of Daily Breathing (see chapter 11, page 151), in which you move your body horizontally along the floor. To loosen your scalp, you move it horizontally over your skull.
- You don't have to choose between Little Circles and Back-and-Forths. You can work a complete area with one and then the other, in whichever order feels right.
- As you're working, note tight areas and sore points and then return to loosen them further.

Back of the Head

Move the back of your scalp using Little Circles or Back-and-Forths.

1. Make Puppy Dog Paws.
2. Bend your forearms up, elbows pointed diagonally in front of you, relax your shoulders, and place both hands at the back of your head.
3. Splay your fingers out into two semicircles, index fingers

together, and place them more or less horizontally across the bottom of your skull, latching on underneath your hair.

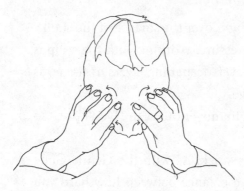

Fig. 17-1. Little Circles along occipital ridge and moving up the back of the head

4. Do Little Circles, with both hands moving together rhythmically in an outward direction. You can follow this with (or substitute it with) Back-and-Forths, moving your scalp up and down in a vertical direction.

5. Begin behind your ears, at the bottom edge of your skull (the "yes-no joint") and work your way up to the occipital ridge, massaging back and forth along the whole lower skull and under and on the ridge. If needed, repeat or focus on particular knots until they feel loosened.

6. Continue up the back of the skull, with fingers held horizontally or vertically — whichever feels best — and both hands circling outward. The idea is to create movement.

7. Once you've reached the top, start again with both hands near the bottom of your skull, working the entire middle swath up to the top of the box.

8. Start again at the bottom, this time with your hands farther apart, so the next swath covers the remainder of the back of the box, out to its sides and top corners.

Sides of the Head

Move the sides of your scalp using Little Circles or Back-and-Forths.

1. Place your hands on either side of your head, with fingers splayed out into a half-circle above your ears; pinkies will be on your hairline in front. Latch on with Little Frog Pads.
2. Do Little Circles, circling toward your face, or Back-and-Forths in an up-down direction. To do both, move hands rhythmically in coordination.

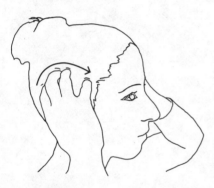

Fig. 17-2. Little Circles up the sides of the head, circling forward

3. Make your way up to the top corners of the sides of the box, pinkies following your hairline.
4. Do one or two more passes, with each pass farther toward the back of your head until your index fingers reach and complete the swath at the back corners of the sides of the box.

Top of the Head

Move the top of your scalp using Little Circles or Back-and-Forths.

1. With your arms bent, elbows in front, palms turned toward your face, and soft hands and fingers, latch your finger pads onto your hairline, under your hair, at the top of your forehead.
2. Separate your fingers to span the width of your forehead at your hairline, with each pinkie on what would be a center part. Your thumbs can join in too.

3. Glide the top of your scalp over your skull using Little Circles, rhythmically moving both hands together in an inward direction.

4. Then do Back-and-Forths in a front-back direction, beginning again at your hairline. With either stroke, your forehead should move. Do the entire top of your skull, inching your way to the back of the top of the box.

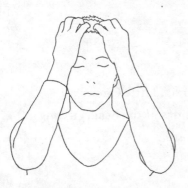

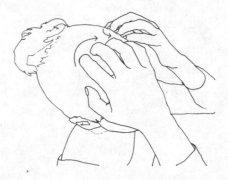

Fig. 17-3a. Little Circles (circling inward) and/or Back-and-Forths, top of the head (front view)

Fig. 17-3b. Little Circles (circling inward), top of the head.

Alternative Back-and-Forths Move

1. Curve your hands and place your fingers back-to-back.
2. Place your fingertips on what would be a middle part in your hair, pinkies at your hairline.
3. Latch on and move your scalp front to back.
4. Then slightly release contact and reposition your fingers, with hands a little farther apart this time.

5. Do Back-and-Forths, and repeat until hands reach both corners of the top of the box. Then reposition them to the next swath back and repeat until they reach the back of the top of the box.

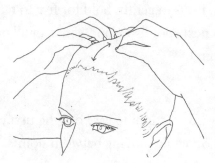

Fig. 17-3c. Back-and-Forths (front-back), top of the head.

Check-In

How does your head feel after massaging your entire scalp? Does it feel tingly and loose? If you had an impending headache, did it shift? Did it begin to subside, or did it get stronger? If needed, return to work on tight, stuck, or sore points until they are relieved.

The Face

If your face feels tight and tired, you deserve to relax and rejuvenate it by giving yourself a face massage. You will again latch onto the surface of the skin, so that you don't pull it, and use the points of contact to go deeper. Palpate for areas and points that are stuck and tight (instead of those that are pulsing and pounding), especially in the forehead, temple, and eye areas — and sometimes the jaw.

In addition to Little Circles, there are three new moves for the face: Press-and-Hold and Pull-Downs are used for most moves on the face; the Channel Stroke is used for the jawline.

Press-and-Hold

Make Puppy Dog Paws and then latch on with Little Frog Pads to the point(s) you are working on. Press in gently, hold for five to ten seconds, release and apply to the next spot using one, some, or all of your fingers as per the instructions.

Pull-Downs

Do Press-and-Hold with downward traction: to ease out the tissue, maintain light contact and traction while moving between points.

The Forehead

Ease and relieve forehead pain, tightness, and constriction; and smooth furrowed brow and frown lines.

1. Bend your arms with elbows forward, palms toward your face, fingers curved, and hands soft.
2. Bring your pinkies together and spread your fingers horizontally. Covering the width of the forehead, latch onto the hairline at the top.
3. Working gently, latch on with just enough contact to move your forehead tissue.
4. Do Little Circles, with each hand circling in an inward direction, the opposite of stretching it taught.
5. Spiral your way down your forehead to the valley just above your brow bone.
6. You can do Pull-Downs in addition to or instead of Little Circles, starting again at the top of the forehead.
7. Identify stuck or tight areas and return to further loosen them if needed.

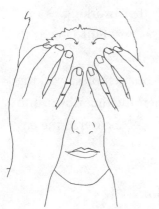

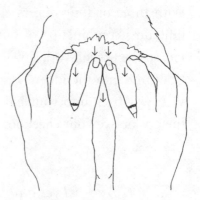

Fig. 17-4. Little Circles, forehead, circling inward

Fig. 17-5. Pull-Downs, forehead

Temples

Release temple and jaw tension and pain, which are often connected to stress, gum chewing, unconscious teeth grinding (bruxism), bite misalignment, and jaw holding and clenching. The temples can be sore and sensitive, so use very gentle touch.

1. Place your fingers on your temples (at the sides of your forehead) along the top diagonal ridge before they dip into the shallow valley of your sphenoid bone.

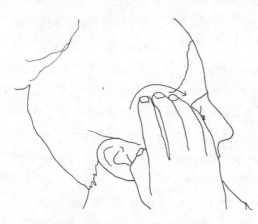

Fig. 17-6. Little Circles, temples, circling toward the face

2. With three or four fingers close together, working as one unit, do a combination of Little Circles and Pull-Downs to loosen the tissue. Work slowly and gently.

3. Continue into the indented area of your temples, working your way back into your hairline, then moving down into the upslope of your cheekbone until you've covered the entire area.

Eyes and Brow Bone

Ease eye-area tension created by stress, straining, squinting, and overuse. This area is delicate, so work on it even more gently. *Note: Do eye massage on the bones that encircle the eye, not on the eyelid or the soft area below the eye.*

1. Work on the top, front, and underside surfaces of the brow bone as if it is a window ledge on a façade (which is your face). Hold each set of points for five to ten seconds.

2. Top: Splay your fingers in a half-circle just above your eyebrows on the upslope of your brow bone. Pinkies are above the bridge of your nose; index fingers fan out to the sides of your eyes on the outside of the brow. Do several Press-and-Holds, Pull-Downs, or a combination of both.

3. Front: Move your fingers down a bit and place them onto your eyebrows, like you're Spider-Man latched onto a building. Your pinkie, ring, and middle fingers will fit into the little indentations along the bone as follows: your pinkies, nearest your nose; ring fingers, above the inside corners of your eyes; middle fingers, at the arches; and index fingers, atop the outer corner of the eye sockets. Apply Press-and-Hold with light pressure straight in.

4. Underside: Place your fingers on the underside of the brow bone, again finding the notches. Straighten your fingers

slightly and apply very gentle pressure with a slight upward traction and hold for five to ten seconds.

5. Outside corner: Use three or four fingers together for Press-and-Holds to the area at the outer corners of the bony eye socket. You can also use slight traction in two separate ways: downward and outward. Breathe.

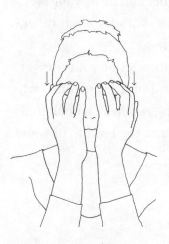

Fig. 17-7a. Top (above eyebrows): Pull-Down

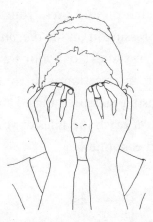

Fig. 17-7b. Front (on eyebrows): Press-and-Hold

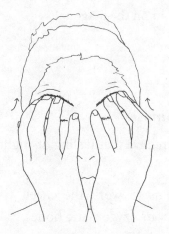

Fig. 17-7c. Underside (below eyebrows): Press-and-Hold, upward traction

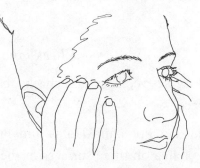

Fig. 17-8. Outside corner (of eye socket): Press-and-Hold

Nose and Sinuses

Release tightness and tenderness adjacent to your nose and cheeks and relieve sinus congestion and pain.

1. Do Press-and-Holds on both sides of your face at once using the pads of your middle fingers.
2. At the slope of your nose next to inner corner of your eyes, latch on and press your middle fingers toward each other, pressing in on the *diagonal* (see fig. 17-9).
3. Press-and-Hold your way down both sides of your nose at its intersection with your cheeks, finding the indentations, using pressures angled straight in and on the diagonal until you reach the sides of your nostrils and the bottom of your cheekbones.

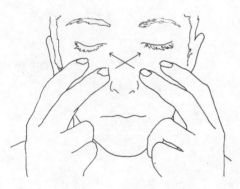

Fig. 17-9. **Press-and-Hold, side of nose/cheek, pressing in on the diagonal**

Cheekbones and Sinuses

Release eye, sinus, and cheek areas, and relieve that feeling of "tight face."

1. Do Press-and-Holds and Pull-Downs to work the cheek area on three surfaces of the cheekbone (zygomatic bone). As with your brow, imagine your face is like a façade with a window ledge (your cheekbone) that has a top, front, and underside.

2. Top: Following the line of the bone, splay three or four fingers in a half-circle in the indentations of your cheekbones and work your way out into your hairline.

3. Front: Place your fingers on the front surface of your cheekbones, fitting your fingers into the indentations on the bone near your nose, and work your way across the arch into your upper jaw.

4. Underside: Slightly straighten your fingers and place them on the underside of the cheekbone near your nose. Again find the indentations, and work your way to your ear.

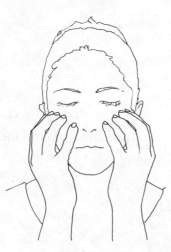

Fig. 17-10. **Cheekbone finger placement**

Jaw and Temporomandibular Joint

Release jaw and head tension due to stress, teeth grinding, jaw clenching, misalignment, and gum chewing.

Your jaw joint, or temporomandibular joint (TMJ), is located directly in front of and about halfway down the length of your ears and is the hinge for your upper jaw (the *maxilla*) and lower jaw (the *mandible*). The muscle that joins them (called the *masseter*) is the strongest in your body according to weight.

1. For jaw massage, start above the hinge and latch on with Little Frog Pads about one inch inside your hairline. Place your

fingers horizontally in the valley of your temporal bone just above your zygomatic arch.

2. Do a combination of Pull-Downs and Little Circles, in either order.

3. Pull-Downs: Press in while exerting slight downward traction. Release traction slightly but not completely, and work your way down in front of your ears to the "pointed corners" of your lower jaw.

4. Little Circles: Go over the same area. At the bottom corner, focus on the indentations on the front surface.

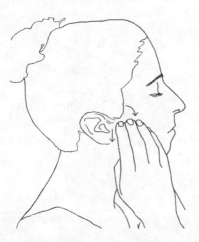

Fig. 17-11. **Pull-Downs and Little Circles around the jaw joint**

Jawline and Chin

Release jaw and head tension and habitual holding due to stress, teeth grinding, jaw clenching, and gum chewing. Jawline and chin release work are done purely on the bone, and *not* farther in under the chin or neck near the glands.

JAWLINE: CHANNEL STROKE
Work your way from the back corner of your jaw down to the chin using Channel Stroke.

1. Fold both index fingers and place them over the bottom corner of your jawbone below the ear, one on each side, and place your thumbs on the underside, forming a channel for your lower jaw.
2. Gently tug the tissue down and forward over the bone with the sides of both index fingers while pressing up and back with your thumbs on the underside of the bone, creating a pinching, twisting-like movement.

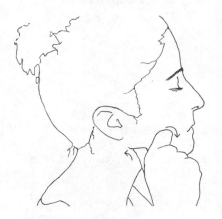

Fig. 17-12. **Channel Stroke along the jawline**

Chin Squeeze

This move releases chin tension, which is often a surprising find.

1. Using your right hand, pinch the right-side corner of your chin between your thumb on the bottom and the side of your folded index finger on top. Latch onto your chin tissue, pulling it down over the bone, and hold and squeeze with your index finger while using your thumb on the bottom of the bone as a fulcrum. As you squeeze, breathe and let go of the holding in your chin. Then release your grip, and repeat a few times.
2. Now move to the middle of your chin. Do the same move: place a crooked index finger over the middle of your chin,

and use the thumb under the bone as a fulcrum. Pull down, squeeze, and let go of your chin tension.

3. Switch hands and repeat on the left side.

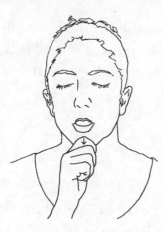

Fig. 17-13. Chin Squeeze

Massage Closing and Assessment

- Gently remove your hands from your face. With your eyes closed, let the treatment settle in.
- Take stock of what has changed and where. How do you feel compared to when you started? How are you now, what do you notice, and where is your headache (if you had one)?
- By knowing how you got to this place of relief, you can better replicate it. Perhaps tomorrow you'll notice your shoulders are tight and then be able to soften them with a squeeze.
- The more you practice, the better you'll feel and the more you'll want to make self-massage a regular habit.
- Shake out your hands and arms mindfully (you can do this throughout your session), to get rid of what you collected.
- Slowly open your eyes.

Don't Test the Treatment!

After a bodywork session, I always tell my clients, "Don't test the treatment!"

Just about everybody tries to stretch up and out of themselves to see if they feel better or looser, or have less pain — including me before I knew better. I call this "testing the treatment." Don't do it.

When you stretch or twist your neck after bodywork, it's counterproductive because you contract the very muscles and fascia that you just relaxed. Instead of pulling your head up and away, let your head settle onto your body.

Next Steps

If you are working with an *active* headache or migraine or specific areas or points of pain (as opposed to doing your prevention routine), your next step is to take an assessment:

- If your headache, migraine, tension, or pain is gone, you can stop here.
- If you still feel tension or pain in specific areas, return to them and do more detailed work.
- If you worked on the back of your neck or lower skull and your headache or migraine has released to the front of your head and is beginning to increase, apply the Mundo Method, which you will learn in the next two chapters.

Upper Body Self-Massage:
Short-Form Instructions
for Easy Reference

After you have learned the details of the techniques in chapters 15, 16, and 17, you can use these instructions as a kind of shorthand. As explained in chapter 16, under "How to Use Self-Massage" (page 216), you can do the entire routine at once, target different areas each day, or zone in on tight or painful areas that are bothering you. No matter which approach you take, always begin with The Basics.

1. THE BASICS

- Align posture; give feet a broad base, toes parallel; breathe into belly; find center.
- Rest tongue on roof of mouth; let teeth slightly part.
- Keep head straight as if looking straight ahead. Don't twist or tilt it up, down, or to the side.
- Let go of all thoughts and close your eyes.
- Warm and soften hands.

2. SHOULDERS

- Warm and loosen shoulders.
- Reach around front to opposite shoulder, keep shoulders down, arm and elbow relaxed on chest.
- Shoulder ridge: Squeeze-and-Hold, continuing down into upper arm.
- Shoulder ridge: Squeeze-Release, continuing down into upper arm.
- Shoulder ridge: Little Circles and/or Back-and-Forths.

3. BACK OF SHOULDER / UPPER BACK

- Squeeze-and-Hold.
- Squeeze-Release.
- Little Circles and/or Back-and-Forths, focusing on scapular ridge and levator scapulae.

4. CHEST

- Upper Chest Taps.
- Openers: sternum and clavicle stretch.
- Spider Silk Pull.

5. BACK OF NECK

- Kitty-Scruff Hold.
- Squeeze-Release.
- Three Strips up the Back of the Neck.

6. SIDES OF NECK

- SCM: Gentle Glide-Release.
- "Bermuda Triangle": Gentle Glide-Release.

7. HEAD

- Approach with care; work under your hair. Latch onto scalp with Little Frog Pads.
- Back of head: Little Circles (outward direction) or Back-and-Forths (vertical direction) on lower skull, occipital ridge, and back of head; work your way up.
- Sides of head: Little Circles (circling toward face) or Back-and-Forths (up and down), fingers splayed horizontally, pinkies on hairline; work your way up.
- Top of head: Little Circles (hands circling toward each other) or Back-and-Forths (front and back direction), palms turned toward face, fingers splayed horizontally on hairline, pinkies side-by-side; work your way back in two or more swaths.
- Top of head: Alternative Back-and-Forths move. Starting with fingers along center part of hair, work both hands out to sides and in swaths to back edge of the top of the box.

8. FACE

- Approach face with even more care. Loosen tissue subtly, palpating for stuck, tight areas.
- Forehead: Splay fingers along hairline, palms toward face, pinkies side by side. Move your way down with Little Circles (inward direction) and Pull-Downs. Separate hands wider and work another swath.
- Temples: Little Circles (toward face) and Pull-Downs.
- Eyes and brow bone: Press-and-Holds on three surfaces of brow and outer corners of eye sockets.

- Nose and sinus points: Press-and-Holds.
- Cheekbones: Press-and-Holds on three surfaces.
- Jaw/TMJ: Little Circles and Pull-Downs.
- Jawline: Channel Stroke.
- Chin: Chin Squeeze.

9. MASSAGE CLOSING AND SELF-ASSESSMENT

10. SHAKE IT OUT!

11. NEXT STEPS: Complete your massage, go back to specific areas for detailed work, or apply the Mundo Method. Refer to "Next Steps" in this chapter; see page 251 for the criteria.

Make an entry in your diary when you do self-massage, including what you do and for how long. Note how you feel afterward: relaxed, softer, tighter, more open, less pain, more pain, sore, tired, energized, headache relieved, headache exacerbated and where. Continue to use these routines as maintenance, even when you are feeling better and no longer recording in your diary.

18 Headaches in the Language of Touch

*A*s a dedicated headache healer, you are now ready to enter the realm of the Mundo Method to relieve your active migraine or tension headache on the spot. This headache touch therapy uses subtle touch and focused concentration to work with specific headache sensations rather than on a fixed anatomical spot. As with the touch therapies you have just learned, it is a dynamic process, like a kind of noninstrumental biofeedback: your real-time responses *during* the treatment will determine each successive area to work on and type of application to use.

In this chapter you will learn what the Mundo Method is all about, including kinesthetic distinctions and markers for different types of headaches, preparatory energy-touch work, mental exercises, and other lessons, including hand placement and "head-mapping." So let's delve into the specially illustrated, fascinating world of Mundo Method concepts, terms, and techniques.

A Headache from the Outside

Naturally, I don't have to tell you how horrible you feel on the *inside* from the disorienting, sick, painful symptoms that overtake your head and entire being when you have a migraine. But you might not know, realize, or believe that you can release your pain's pulsing, pounding, stuck sensations by locating and working *with* them from the *outside*.

Like touch, headaches have a subtle language all their own, which you can learn by listening with your hands. But what exactly do you listen for, and how can you tell if you have found it? And are all headache types alike?

Headache Types Are Unique

Each headache type has particular qualities and involves distinct sensations. Therefore, the touch therapy protocol you will be using will depend on the type of headache you have at the time.

Tension-Type Headache Feels Stuck and Tight

- These headaches feel stuck, tight, and band-like, like a too-tight hatband or a vise. They don't move or pulse strongly.
- There is a generalized tightness, a contracted, seized-up quality to the scalp, head, face, neck, shoulders, chest, and arms.
- Tension-type headaches are located in the forehead, the temples, around the eyes and nose, and around the circumference of the head.
- A knot, or stuck spot, can be present in the back of the neck, lower skull, jaw, upper back, and/or shoulders.

Protocol: First loosen and release the shoulders, neck, head, and face with self-massage; then you can follow with a brief Mundo Method application to balance the head.

Migraine Feels Pulsing and Electrical

- Migraines have a pulsatile quality, with more amplitude, or strength, than a regular pulse.
- There is often an electrical quality, like mini-explosions on the head.
- Migraines are located in the forehead and temples (and into the hairline) on one or both sides; also around the eyes, nose, and jaw.
- More rarely, migraine involves other points located at or near the top of the head in either front quadrant.

Protocol: Apply the Mundo Method to quiet or still all pulsing and/or painful headache points until migraine is released.

Migraine with Tension Headache Symptoms Feels Both Pulsing and Stuck

- Qualities of both types are combined: pulsing, pounding, electrical — and stuck, tight, seized, contracted.
- Stuck, tight, tension headache components cover over, or hold down, migraine pulsations like a snug cap.
- When tension headache is released, migraine is uncovered.
- This type of headache can (and often does) include the presence of a knot, or stuck spot, in the back of the neck, lower skull, upper back, and/or shoulders.
- Releasing the headache from stuck areas in the back makes it "bloom" in the front of the head, yielding more specific points to work on.

Protocol: *First*, gently loosen and release stuck, tight areas in the neck, shoulders, scalp, and face with self-massage to help the migraine shift to the front of the head; *then* apply the Mundo Method.

Migraine Variations That Feel Generalized and Difficult to Pinpoint

These variations are named for their qualities.

- Watery
  - o Diffuse pain
  - o Temples feel tender and puffy to the touch as if retaining water

- Not fully descended
  - o Diffuse quality and difficult to locate both on the inside and the outside of the head
  - o All over and nowhere at the same time
  - o Challenging to know where to apply touch therapy
  - o As if on the verge of a migraine throughout the whole body; constantly impending

Protocol: Pick a spot, any spot. Apply Mundo Method with exceptionally light touch to all pulsing points until migraine is released. If needed, first use self-massage with minimal movement, and very light touch, to release any stuck points.

Mundo Method Concepts

These concepts introduce you to working with your headaches using body and mind.

Locate the Headache with Your Touch

You must first locate the headache in a specific spot on your head in order to work on it.

- When you as the therapist locate the headache on the outside with your touch, you will often find that what seemed

from the inside like overall pain is actually the sum of multiple distinct points.

- Whether your pain is generalized, in one spot, or in several,
  you release it by working on one point at a time.

Spider Push-Ups on a Mirror

A riddle from my childhood will help you locate your headache.
Do the moves pictured below by putting your fingers together and
moving them in and out. Here's the riddle: What's this?

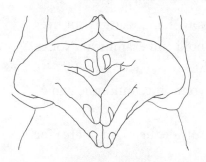
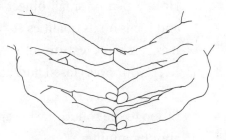

Fig. 18-1a. Spider Push-Ups on a
Mirror, fingers extended position

Fig. 18-1b. Spider Push-Ups on a
Mirror, fingers together position

Answer: A spider doing push-ups on a mirror!

Your forehead is like the mirror in the riddle. It serves as the
point of contact between the inside and outside of your head. The
spider legs are like your touch; you match your touch with the sensations you feel both outside your head (as the massage therapist)
and inside your head (as the headache sufferer). You experience
pain on the inside and come along on the outside with your touch,
matching it directly to your pain's location.

Even if your pain moves, you follow and match it with your
touch. The advantage of working on your own headache is that
you can locate your pain on the inside because you can usually tell

where it hurts. The downside is that you have to work on yourself while you're in pain.

Move into *the Pain with Touch and Awareness*

With the Mundo Method, you move *into* the heart of the pain. Although you might feel like you want to numb it or run away, if you stay present and work on it, physically and mentally, you can shift it.

MIND FOCUS EXERCISE

This exercise illustrates the power of your mental focus.

1. Hold a pen or small object in your hand. Close your eyes and focus on its qualities as you hold and examine it. Notice its size, shape, texture, and weight.
2. Keep your eyes closed and hold your object until the end of the exercise.
3. Listen to the sounds inside and outside the room or area for about a minute.
4. Next recall what you had for breakfast.
5. Then open your eyes and put down your object.
6. Debrief:

    *   What did you notice about your pen or object?
    *   What happened to the pen when you listened for sounds?
    *   What happened to the sounds when you remembered breakfast?
    *   What happened to thoughts of breakfast when you refocused on the pen?
    *   Did you notice that when your attention was elsewhere, its former subject seemed to fade into the background — and what you *now* attended to became stronger?

    It's as if your attention is like a channel selector that amplifies whatever you focus on. Indeed, when you use your channel selector to focus on your pain as you work on it, you will get more information, be more effective, and feel when it shifts.

Approach Your Head and Face with Care

Your head and face are delicate, and when you have a migraine, they often become hypersensitive to touch, a symptom called *allodynia*.

- When you go to touch your head, enter into its surrounding field gently, as if you're dipping your toes into water to test the temperature.
- Less is more. You don't want to jostle anything.

The Process Is Similar to Fixing a Broken Circuit or Plumbing Line

The overall concept of the method is about restoring flow.

- When you fix a broken circuit or pipe, you restore the connection so the electricity or water can flow through.
- Do you remember as a kid pulling a horseshoe magnet through the sandbox and seeing the iron filings align to its poles? Similarly, applying the Mundo Method is like repairing a break in a line, or magnetizing the iron filings in a sandbox — but in your head: You cause the energy to flow in the same direction, in this case, from front to back.
- When you quiet the out-of-control volatility of the headache, its jangly energy organizes, flow is restored, and its pain is released.

Loosen What's Tight, Still What's Pulsing (or Do Both in That Order)

The type of headache you're having determines which protocol to use:

- For tension headache, loosen tight, stuck areas with self-massage.
- For migraine, still or quiet its pulsations with the Mundo Method.
- If you have symptoms of both types at once, first loosen, then still.

Headaches Can Move

Your headache or migraine might start on one side then move to the other.

- For example, it begins in your left temple, and as you work on it, it moves to a different point on that side or even to the other temple.
- Headaches can seem like entities unto themselves. Sometimes it's as if you have to chase them around and corner them like little gophers!

Release All the Pulsing Points

As you work on one headache point and release it, the next point (if there's more than one) will come to the fore.

- Stay with it, and keep finding your way into each painful point to release it.
- You have to release all the pulsing points for the overall headache to release!

The Cycle Must Complete!

As the headache releases and resolves, a palpable set of changes occurs, both on the inside of your head, where you feel less pain, and on the outside, where you can feel the headache release with your hands.

- The sensations of the release are different than those of the headache itself.
- You must feel the release! In order for the headache cycle to complete and the pain to subside, you must feel the release of headache sensations in your hands. This process will be covered in chapter 19.

Mundo Method Terms and Techniques

The metaphor "doing geography on your head" aptly describes the Mundo Method terms and techniques that show how to determine the placement of both hands in relation to your headache.

The Head Is Like a Globe

Think of your head as a globe — after all, it is basically shaped like one.

- You will be working on your head as if it's a globe, applying the Mundo Method around its circumference and straight through its diameter.

Front and Back of the Head

What are the "front and back" of the head, and how do you determine them along with placement of your "giving and receiving hands," a.k.a. "front and back hands"? And what are those, anyway?

- One hand always works with the headache in front (the front hand) while the other hand is placed on the back of your head (the back hand).
- To delineate the front and back of your head:
  - o Place your head level, eyes forward, checking that your chin isn't tilted up or down.

- o Touch the top point of your ears with your index fingers and then draw a vertical line straight up the sides of your head until both fingers meet at the top.
- o That imaginary line divides your head into front and back.
- Everything in front of the line is called the *front* of the head; everything in back of the line is called the *back* of the head.
- One hand (the front hand) always works with the headache in front while the other hand (the back hand) is placed on the back of the head.

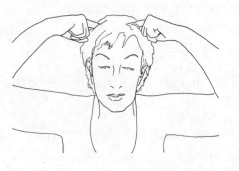

Fig. 18-2. **Dividing the front and back of the head**

Work from the Front to the Back of the Head

Now that we've defined the front and back of the head, and front and back hands, here's how to use those distinctions:

- Always work from the front to the back of the head: apply the Mundo Method by working with and releasing the headache in front and then receiving its sensations in back.
- However, if the headache feels stuck in the back of your neck or lower skull, first do self-massage to release it to the front. This move also makes a diffuse-seeming migraine become stronger and more defined in front, which makes it easier to pinpoint and work on. Then apply the Mundo Method.

Your Hands Work 180 Degrees Apart

Position your hands 180 degrees apart from each other at the circumference of your head. (Think of the earth's equator on a globe.) Your hands will be opposite each other — and work in conjunction.

- Always place one hand on the left side, or hemisphere (as in left and right brain hemispheres), of your head, and the other hand on the right side of your head.
- Because your hands are working 180 degrees apart, one hand will always be working on the headache in front of the front-back dividing line, and one will always be working in back of that dividing line — *and* in opposite hemispheres.
- The hands are never placed front to front or back to back, meaning both hands will never work in front or in back of the dividing line, or on the same side or hemisphere, at the same time. For example, if your right thumb is working on a headache point on your right temple, you would position your left palm directly opposite it — on the left hemisphere at the back of your head. You can trace a line between them, up and over, as if you're flying a polar route.
- When your front hand moves to another headache point, your back hand moves too, if needed, in order to maintain that half-circle distance.

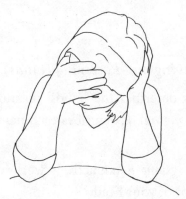

Fig. 18-3. Mundo Method, thumb on right temple, palm on back left quadrant

Occipital Ridge Position

The hand at the back of your head is always placed on or above the occipital ridge, not on your lower skull or neck.

- To find the occipital bone and ridge: Place your palm on the flat area of the back of your head and find the sloping ridge at the bottom edge of your skull. Run your fingers along the ridge to palpate it. It feels like a rocky overhang, below which the bottom of your skull drops off and slopes in toward your neck.
- Always position your front and back hands at the same height. Using the metaphor of "geography on your head," they would be at the same latitude — in other words, not on the front of your head and the back of your neck. I often explain it as: you're working straight through the brain.

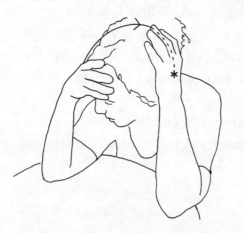

Fig. 18-4. **Back hand placement, from thumb in the front, over "North Pole," to middle of palm at back of your head**

Front and Back Hands (or Giving and Receiving Hands)

The phrase *front and back hands* describes the hands' positioning on the head. *Giving and receiving hands* describes each hand's function.

- The *front hand*, also called the *giving hand*, actively works with your headache on the front of your head.

- The *back hand*, also called the *receiving hand*, has a more passive job of receiving the headache when it releases to the back.
- Hands are termed *front* and *back*, instead of *right* and *left*, because you'll use the hand on the same side that your headache is on:
  - If your headache is on the left, you'll use your left hand to work on it in front.
  - If it's on your right, you'll use your right hand in front.
  - Therefore, which hand is the front, or giving, hand will depend on the location of the headache point you're working on. (If you tried to use the hand on the opposite side of your headache, instead of the same side, you'd have to torque your neck to get both hands in position.)

The Back Hand's Special Role

The back, or receiving, hand plays an essential role. It completes the "break in the line" and helps reestablish flow. Yet its role is passive and receptive, as illustrated by the following analogy:

Imagine that you're teaching a class, and a teacher friend has arrived early to meet you for lunch. She is waiting patiently at the back of the room. You know she's there, but you're not paying attention to her because you're teaching.

Your friend is like the back hand. You don't engage with her until you're done teaching.

- In the Mundo Method, your receiving hand rests lightly on the back of your head.
- You know it's there, waiting, but you're not focused on it — that is, not until your headache starts to release in the front and the back hand's role is activated.

Giving and Receiving Hands Exercise

This preparatory exercise demonstrates the concepts and experience of the giving and receiving hands and moving a headache with your mind. It builds on the Energize Your Hands touch prep exercise in chapter 15 (see page 204).

1. Close your eyes during this exercise. Make Puppy Dog Paws, then energize your hands by firmly pressing your palms together and rubbing them briskly until warmed.

2. Place your hands face-up on your lap and bring your awareness into both palms. Use your mind to focus on them.

3. Now focus your attention on your right palm, then your left, and repeat the focus rhythmically: right left, right left, right left, right left. In this case, your right hand is *giving*, and your left is *receiving*.

4. Now reverse the order. (Reenergize your hands, if needed.) Focus on your left palm, then your right. Use your attention to repeat the focus rhythmically: left right, left right, left right, left right. In this case, your left hand is *giving*, and your right is *receiving*.

5. By reversing the order of your focus, you reversed their roles.

6. Now reverse it again: right left, right left, right left, right left.

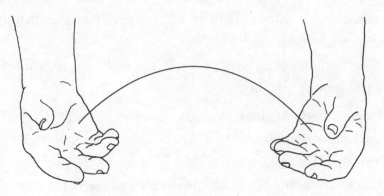

Fig. 18-5. Giving and Receiving Hands

Isn't that interesting? You changed the direction of energy flow in your hands with your mind. What did you feel? Did you notice sensations of warmth, pulsation, or tingling jump from your right to your left hand and then switch directions when you changed the order of your attention? Focusing your mind on the sensations you feel in your hands and directing your mental energy is a key Mundo Method technique.

Communication Pathways

By using touch and concentration to work on your headache pain, you set up multiple communication pathways.

- Your hands communicate with your head to palpate and manipulate sensations and pain.
- Your hands communicate with each other to gauge their relative positioning, their next moves, and the timing of their specific functions.
- Your focused concentration is the glue in those communications.

Mundo Method therapy is different than a purely physical application of pressure to the temples, after which headache pain typically returns. Along with subtle manipulation of sensations, the focused concentration component helps to restore flow and break the cycle by occupying, releasing, and recycling the headache.

Stilling a Migraine

Stilling is the technique at the heart of the Mundo Method. It helps you calm your headache using subtle pressure distinctions and focused concentration. To release each painful point on the front of the head, you must Still, or quiet, it, both physically and mentally.

The physical portion is called *Flattening*. Flattening a migraine is different than self-massage, where you loosen and ease into layers of tight tissue and create movement. In migraine especially, you want to calm the area instead because any movement would add another rhythm and produce more pain.

The *Mental Push* is the focused concentration (mental) component of the Mundo Method. It is the most esoteric and revolutionary of the hands-on techniques I teach because it uses the power of your mind to move your pain. It speeds up the process and reduces the amount of physical pressure needed, so you don't inadvertently use too much, the typical mistake made by headache healers in training.

Flattening and Amplitude

Migraines (and tension headaches to a lesser degree) are typically made up of one or several pulsing points, some weaker and some stronger. Imagine a sound wave mapped on an oscilloscope. The height of the wave, or amplitude, will be taller or shorter depending on the sound's volume. Brain-wave states are also characterized by their amplitude and frequency and can be detected by electrodes placed on the scalp and then measured and recorded during a test called an *electroencephalogram* (EEG), or during EEG biofeedback, also called *neurofeedback*.

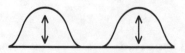
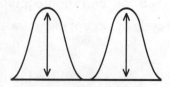

Lower amplitude   **Higher amplitude**
Quieter   **Louder**
Milder headache pulsation **Stronger headache pulsation**

Fig. 18-6. Sound wave demonstrating headache amplitude

The amplitude of a headache point correlates to the strength of the pulsation in that point. The amount of pressure needed in order to Flatten it depends on its amplitude, or pulsation strength. In other words, what would it take to make the wave flat? When the pain is more marked, it seems to have higher amplitude and jump out of your head. A milder headache with lower amplitude would take less pressure to Flatten than a migraine with higher amplitude, which would need slightly more.

Note: When I say *pressure*, I mean *extremely light* touch. This light: Place your palms on a table or desk without pressing. Simply place them. That's how light.

As your self-massage routine moved from shoulders to face, you used successively lighter pressure to accommodate the delicateness of tissue. Your headache needs the lightest pressure yet because you're working with pulsations, not tissue quality. To pick up the earlier metaphor of squeezing fruit to test for its ripeness: Some people squeeze produce so hard that they make a dent that will bruise it. That squeeze uses too much pressure. Same goes for treating migraine. The Flattening technique will help you gauge how much is just right to dismiss your headache pain.

The Flattening Technique

Here's how to Flatten an active migraine or tension headache (use this technique with step 8 of the Mundo Method Self-Care Instructions, chapter 19, page 285):

1. Match your touch to a painful point, as you did in Spider Push-Ups on a Mirror.
2. With your touch, listen for the amplitude, or pulsation strength, of the painful point.
3. Flatten each pulsing, painful point using light pressure,

while focusing on it mentally with the Mental Push (see next section).

4. Use *only* the amount of physical pressure it takes to Flatten the wave at its own level of amplitude; meet the pulsation with your touch and Flatten it to make it flush with your head.

   - *Use very light touch.*
   - The hand-over-fist image in figure 18-7a is a representation of your forehead and your headache. The hand represents your forehead. The fist represents your headache, pulsing and pounding from the inside of your head and pushing against it.
   - Try it! Cover your fist with your other palm and pulse your fist against your palm as if it's your headache.

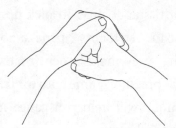

Fig. 18-7a. The headache (fist) pulsating in your forehead (palm)

5. When you come along from the outside with your touch, match your touch to the headache's amplitude or strength of pulsation.

   - Too much pressure would make the pulsing point concave as in the second image (18-7b).

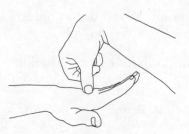

Fig. 18-7b. Too much pressure (thumb) on a painful point (back of hand) makes the headache pulsation concave.

- And oppositely, insufficient pressure would let the pulsation push into your fingers or thumb instead of Flattening it.

6. With just the right pressure (as in the third image, 18-7c), the pulsation is made flush, or even, with your head, instead of it pushing your thumb out. In each moment for each headache point, use the amplitude and strength of its sensations to gauge the amount of pressure needed.

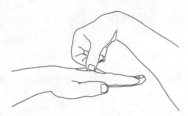

Fig. 18-7c. Use only the amount of pressure needed (thumb) to Flatten the pulsation at its own level of amplitude (back of hand).

Because the physical pressure remains extremely subtle and light, it's the Mental Push that holds the power.

The Mental Push

To do the Mental Push, you focus your mind on the point you are Flattening physically and Still, or quiet, it mentally. It doesn't just happen; you have to make an effort using your mind. Unlike passive volition in biofeedback, the Mental Push involves *active volition* because it is produced by using your will. It's termed a *push* because it requires the mental equivalent of the physical strength used in lifting weights or pushing a piece of heavy furniture across the floor — or imagine the momentum it takes to turn a ship around.

If you've watched Olympic weight lifters on TV or someone pressing two hundred pounds at the gym — or if you yourself have lifted or pushed something heavy, like a couch or car — then you've seen or experienced a *mental push*. More than brute force alone, moving so much weight takes single-minded focus (often accompanied by grunting). At the gym, you wouldn't see someone chatting away, shooting the breeze — as in, "Hey, how you doin'? What's goin' on?" — while lifting heavy weights. Moving heavy weight in gravity doesn't lend itself well to multitasking; anything short of complete focus won't do the job.

How to Do the Mental Push

In the Mental Push you use your mind to help stop your headache and migraine by mentally occupying that point of pain.

FOCUS

Focus your attention on the headache point you're working on Flattening.

- Maintain a neutral state of mind: free of thoughts, distractions, moods, or emotions.
- If your mind wanders, even to wonder about what you're doing, refocus it. Just be with and listen to the sensations.

GATHERING BASKET

Gather your mental energy in your forehead about an inch above your brows, in the triangular area between your eyes. This area is known as an energy center, or chakra, called the third eye.

- In the Mundo Method, I call this space your *Gathering Basket*: the place where you gather your mental energy and from which your Mental Push originates.
- To give your Gathering Basket a trial run, push against something heavy, like your desk or couch, and really try to move it — or just *think* about pushing something heavy. Where does the force of that mental strain originate? Your Gathering Basket!

Depositing the Mental Push

Now take all that concentrated mental energy in your Gathering Basket and push it right into your headache, focusing your mind directly on the point that you're Flattening.

- *In other words, match your touch and your attention with your pain, using the Mental Push to fully occupy it.*

Superhero Attitude

Assume your best superhero attitude. It takes the extraordinary strength of a superhero to dominate the pain of a migraine. Taking on that superhero attitude is what supercharges the Mental Push.

- Think of your favorite hero — one who possesses superhuman strength, a powerful presence, and an unyielding stance.
- Who is it? Wonder Woman? Superman? Nobody wants to risk the consequences of challenging that kind of toughness.
- You need that kind of attitude.

Headache Litany

The Headache Litany is where your superhero takes charge: it's you or your migraine!

The Headache Litany is an internal dialogue that you say to yourself, adopting your best superhero persona, as part of the Mental Push.

Just like an athlete, you must be determined. You can't let worry, doubt, or your opponents get into your head. Those challengers are your headache trying to dominate, and you must say No! So psych yourself up, and do what you've always wanted to do: tell your headache where to go, using your variation of the litany below (adding your own expletives, if you wish).

- Say your litany like a command. Do it like a champion, with authority and righteous indignation, but not with anger, which will only make you tight and reactive. Own it with your hero power, out to save the day for those in need. And guess what? That's you.

- Say your superhero litany in your mind, directing your Mental Push right into the headache point you're Flattening with your touch.

- Ready? Here we go: "Hey, you [fill in the blank] migraine, I'm here now, and guess what? You are *out of here*! I am not taking this anymore! I mean it! You are out of here! Get out! *Out!*"

- To clarify further:

  o You are not trying to push your headache out of that particular point, nor are you trying to move it to the back of your head. Instead, you are pushing your own mind *into* the headache and fully occupying its space, forcing it to go elsewhere (to the back), where it is "recycled."

  o The Mundo Method Self-Care Instructions in chapter 19 will walk you through exactly what to do when each headache point releases in the front of the head.

Re-up

Then what? A headache, especially migraine, is like a recalcitrant child who keeps kicking the seat-back. Just because you ask the child to cut it out doesn't make it happen. If you are repeatedly ignored after several warnings, you might look directly into the child's eyes and say, "I mean it! I said, stop!" *That's* the Re-up.

You have to keep claiming your ground, which in this case, is the headache point that you're Flattening. But a stubborn migraine doesn't just give up and leave with its tail between its legs. It fights back. That's when you Re-up.

"Oh, yeah, you think you're so tough. You can't beat me! I said, you are out of here! Stop! No! I mean it. You're out of here. Get out!"

Re-upping means you keep refocusing your Mental Push, your resolve, in each moment. You have to occupy and conquer each headache point both physically and mentally until the pain dissipates in that spot.

19

Mundo Method Therapy
Self-Care Instructions

*I*n this chapter we put everything together into a routine. You will integrate the information, skills, practices, and distinctions you've learned in the rest of part 4 to work on your own headaches using the Mundo Method. Never before published, these self-care instructions are laid out step by step to make them easy to follow.

Additional techniques and their nuances are detailed and illustrated within the chapter narrative so as not to disrupt the flow of the numbered instructions. You will be ultimately prepared with the final specifics needed to apply the Mundo Method, including a language of sensations when palpating the head, headache, and headache release; body-positioning basics; and instructions for subtly moving between different headache points and for completing the treatment.

Palpating Heads and Headaches:
The Language of Headache Sensations

Now that you know *how* to listen with your touch and concentration and Still the headache physically and mentally, this section focuses on particular qualities of the head, the headache, and the release, describing more precisely *what* to listen for, on your head and in your hands. (You might even experience your own variations.)

You can listen for all of these qualities and sensations. However, to complete the cycle you only need to feel one or a few of the headache and release qualities listed below. With migraine, sensations will typically be more pronounced.

Feel Your Head

Notice how your head feels overall.

- Scalp and forehead: tight, loose
- Tissue quality: alive, dead; present, absent, nobody home; juicy, not juicy
- Tissue or bone: hard, pliable
- Sutures (where your skull bones adjoin): rigid, squared; scalp or forehead tightly seized; skull forms corners
- Overall sense of movement: stuck, still, immobile; loose, pliable, mobile

Listen (with Your Hands) for Pulsations of the Headache

- Location: find the pulsation
- Unilateral or bilateral: pulsation on one side; on both sides; on both sides but pain stronger on one side; starts on one side and moves to the other
- Amplitude: pulsation strong or weak (at each painful point or the headache overall)
- Frequency: pulsation fast or slow
- Beat: pulsation rhythmic or irregular

Various Qualities of Headaches When Palpated

These are qualities and sensations you might feel in each headache point or overall.

- Pulsatile, yet feels stronger and has more amplitude than a regular pulse
- Electrical quality, like mini-explosions on the head
- Intense or weak: how strong the sensations feel to the touch
- Pronounced or subtle; marked, sharp; dull, muted
- Stationary or moving: remains in one place or moves around
- Held down by overall tightness or throbbing, pulsing, pounding
- "Not fully descended," generalized, and all over the place — or "fully blossomed" and concentrated in one or multiple points
- "Watery," puffy as if retaining water

Qualities of the Release

Here are qualities and sensations that come into your back/receiving hand as the headache releases in front. These feel different than the sensations of the headache itself.

- Heat or warmth
- Pulsations, with a regular rhythm or beat
- Slow waves, very slow pulsations, like the vibrational sounds of a gong or bell: "wonnng, wonnng"
- Electrical sensations, like low-grade electrical current
- Twitching, like a twitch with a regular rhythm; located in a specific spot in your palm
- "Wiry" or nervous, like little, irregular twitches
- Magnetic pull; hand feels stuck like a magnet to the back of the head
- Fast or slow: the speed of any sensations that have a beat or rhythm
- Sharp or dull: sensations feel sharp and pronounced or dull and muted
- Intensity: qualities and sensations feel strong or weak
- Empties out all at once or slowly

Basic Body Position

The body positions described in this chapter are designed specifically so you can self-apply the therapy while your head, neck, arms,
hands, and the rest of your body remain relaxed and neutral, not
torqued. Each position is designed to keep your arms from getting tired while your hands stay supported, mobile, relaxed, and
receptive.

While you are learning the Mundo Method, use the basic "Oy,
I've Got Such a Headache" position, described here. After you have
learned this position, you can switch to the reclining body positions
shown later in the chapter (see page 290).

The "Oy, I've Got Such a Headache" Position

This is the basic body position and the easiest one to use when
you're first learning the hands-on therapy. Here a table supports
your elbows; your arms and hands support your head.

1. Sit in a straight-backed chair, feet hip-distance apart, legs
    perpendicular to the floor or extended out slightly.
2. Place both elbows on the table or desk and place your front
    and back hands on your head.

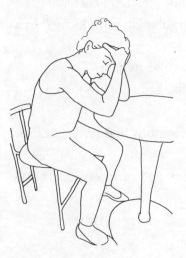

Fig. 19-1a. "Oy, I've Got Such a
Headache" position, elbows on
table

3. Let your upper body bend at the waist and lean over the table at a forty-five-degree angle, so your head falls into your front hand and your neck is relaxed. Situate your chair at the distance from the table that allows your upper torso to be at forty-five degrees.

Mundo Method Self-Care Instructions

This is where you put it all together to relieve your headache pain on the spot.

The instructions are written in short form, so you can refer to them more easily. Use the techniques and information you learned in the rest of part 4, especially chapter 18, to support each step, and refer to them as needed.

Whenever possible, apply the therapy sooner rather than later, just as you would with any acute medication or therapy. It's usually easier to abort a migraine if you can catch it before it escalates or becomes entrenched.

1. Position your body either sitting and leaning over a desk or table, sitting on a couch or in bed with knees up, or lying down in semifetal pose. Use the desk position when you are first learning or away from home without a place to recline or lie down.
2. Loosen any stuck, tight, painful areas in the lower skull, neck, forehead, or jaw with self-massage until the headache shifts to the front of the head. Skip this step if headache or migraine is solely in front.
3. Place both elbows on the table, so your arms don't get tired from being held up, and keep them there during treatment. It's relaxing to let the table hold you up.
4. Make Puppy Dog Paws and drape (don't press) your front hand gently across your forehead, thumb extended. Use the

hand on the same side that your headache is on: right hand on right-sided headache; left hand on left-sided headache. Relaxing the back of your neck, let your head fall into your front hand in the "Oy! I've Got Such a Headache" position. Your arm, hand, and thumb will make a *Y* shape, like a tree trunk and branches, that holds your head up.

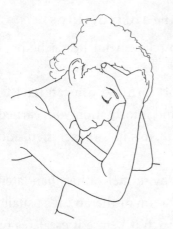

Fig. 19-1b. "Oy, I've Got Such a Headache" position, close-up

5. Find the headache in front: Use the pad of your thumb (your thumbprint) to find your pain by listening for pulsations and other sensations. Remember, you must first locate each headache point in order to work with it. Use your thumb instead of your fingers, so your neck doesn't get twisted when placing your back hand (see step 6).

    Note: Pressing too hard makes it difficult to locate the pulsing point. However lightly you think you're pressing, lighten the pressure once, and then again. Then listen.

6. Lightly position your cupped back hand on the back of your head, with your palm on or above the occipital ridge, not your neck. Place the center of your palm approximately 180 degrees from the headache point that you're working on in front. The back hand should be relaxed and receptive, barely touching your hair, with your attention lightly aware of it.

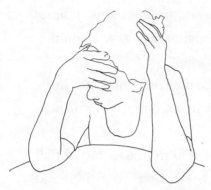

Fig. 19-2. Mundo Method close-up from a different position

7. With your front-hand thumb, attend to and Flatten each pulsing, sore, or aching point, one at a time.

8. Still, or quiet, each headache point in front by Flattening it with your touch and occupying it mentally using the Mental Push. Use very light touch: only the amount of physical pressure it takes to Flatten the pulsation or sensation at its own level of amplitude (see chapter 18, pages 270–71).

9. As the headache begins calming in the point you are working on, let your back hand come into your awareness. Notice if there is a synchronicity between your hands (which you learned to sense in the Giving and Receiving Hands exercise in chapter 18, page 268).

10. As each headache point is "released," notice any sensations that come into your back hand, such as heat, tingling, electricity, waves, slow pulsing, or a magnetic pull. Keep both hands in place. (See Qualities of the Release, this chapter, page 281.)

11. Shift your full attention to the sensations in your back hand. Notice when they subtly begin to *increase* in intensity, keeping your attention on them and whatever you are feeling.

12. Then notice when the sensations in your back hand subtly begin to *subside*.

13. Both the increase and the decrease in sensations indicate that the headache point is shifting, releasing, or beginning to release, and the cycle is completing.

14. Work on all headache points. Use the Directional and Inchworm Techniques (see the following section) to locate and move between them.

15. After the sensations have subsided in front and back for all headache points, remove your hands from your head and keep your eyes closed.

16. "Let the treatment settle in." (I tell this to my clients each time.) Don't test it by moving your head around or stretching your neck from side to side to see if anything has changed. You don't want to jostle anything. Remain peaceful and still. Keep letting the shift settle in and your equilibrium return to normal. Breathe into your belly and allow your head and entire system to rebalance for a minute or so.

17. When you feel ready, open your eyes.

18. This completes one application, which can take from five minutes to an hour, depending on the headache. A severe migraine could take a few one-hour treatments.

19. Notice how you feel: Is your headache gone, shifting and fading away, or still present? If it's still present, has it changed in quality or moved? How and where is it now?

20. If your pain has shifted and lessened, it will usually continue to subside until it's gone. It's as if it has turned a corner. In this case, the treatment is complete.

21. Shake out your hands gently (without jostling your head in the process), until they no longer feel tired, and get rid of what you've collected. (Do this anytime during the treatment if they feel tired or filled up.)

22. If your headache continues or immediately returns after

taking away your hands, repeat the instructions on any re-maining points and areas.

Directional and Inchworm Techniques: Moving from Point to Point

An overall headache or migraine is often made up of closely related painful points, some mere millimeters apart, that seem to mirror trigeminal nerve pathways. Use the Directional and Inchworm Techniques to find and navigate between them.

Directional Technique

Headache points are minute compared to the size of your thumb, so even a slight directional shift of pressure made without lifting a digit can land you on a different point. The Directional Technique helps you zero in on and refine your point of contact.

You can practice the technique on the back of your hand:

1. Place your left palm on your lap with the tip of your right index finger on the back of your left hand.
2. Without lifting your finger, rotate your right hand and your finger a few times slowly in a circle, and notice all the different points you make contact with on your finger and the back of your hand.
3. Now without lifting your finger, slide it away from and toward you, and side to side, keeping it latched onto the surface of your skin. Notice that your finger was still latched onto the same point of skin, yet it made contact with different areas of tissue underneath.

When you use the Directional Technique on your head, each of those minute points of contact could contain a headache. You can often uncover the next point by simply shifting your thumb's direction of pressure on the point you just relieved.

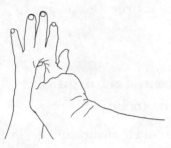

Fig. 19-3. Directional Technique, practiced on back of hand

Inchworm Technique

Make like an inchworm to get from one headache point to another. Practice the technique on the back of your hand, as you did the Directional Technique.

1. Place your left palm on your lap again. Extend your right index finger and place it on the back of your hand just below your wrist.
2. Move your finger as if you are an inchworm, inching your way down your hand to your fingers.
3. When using the Inchworm Technique on your head, once you've found the next point, remain on it. Then follow Mundo Method Instructions to Still it.

When you inch along, your hands remain in contact with your head, and you can find points you might not have noticed had you jumped around to different areas in search of them.

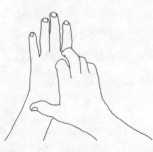

Fig. 19-4a. Inchworm Technique, practiced on back of hand

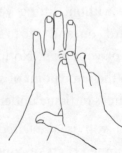

Fig. 19-4b. Inchworm Technique, practiced on back of hand

How the Cycle Completes

"The cycle must complete" means that you have to feel the sensations of the release come into your back hand, feel them intensify, and *then* feel them subside in order for the headache to stop. The release can occur in one of these three different ways:

1. With *each* headache point that you relieve in front, you can feel sensations come into your back hand; it's a one-to-one ratio. And sometimes, there's just one point in front, so you feel the release, and your pain lifts.
2. You have to Still *several* headache points in front before you can feel any sensations come into your back hand.
3. You have to Still, or quiet, *every single* headache point in front before you can feel any sensations come into your back hand.

If you don't feel the release in the back, it means that the cycle has not completed. To remedy this, you have to work on any remaining headache points until you feel the release occur in one of the three ways described. (Also see Qualities of the Release, page 281, and Mundo Method Self-Care Instructions, page 283, both in this chapter.)

Putting It All Together

Putting all the concepts, steps, terms, and techniques together, here's a synopsis of what you're doing in the Mundo Method:

Match your touch to your pain and use the Mental Push to occupy the spot you are gently Flattening with your thumb. Assume a superhero attitude and repeat your Headache Litany in your mind as you work on each headache point, and Re-up mentally to eliminate the pushback. Work on a point until your headache sensations ease in front, release into your back hand, increase in the back, and then subside.

Work on all the pulsing or painful points. As your pain begins to lift, your associated symptoms will also subside. Look for other changes, such as feeling more relaxed, calmer, lighter, hungry, sleepy (if you haven't slept), energetic (if you have), alert, and clear-headed.

Reclining Body Positions

Depending on where you are when a migraine strikes, you can improvise positions in addition to the basic position described above (see page 282). You can also use props! Use pillows or cushions to support your sacrum, arms, and head.

Semi-reclining Position: Couch or Bed

Try this position if you feel up to reclining on your couch or leaning against your headboard. In this position, your knees or thighs serve as your table. (This position is also handy to use when absolutely necessary while seated in a bathroom stall or on a dressing room bench; in these cases, you can modify your positioning slightly with your feet on the floor and your thighs supporting your elbows.)

1. Lean against the back of a couch or a headboard. If the seat is too soft and you sink down, place a pillow under you.
2. Bend your knees, put your feet flat on the bed or couch, and rest both elbows on your knees or thighs. If the couch isn't deep enough to comfortably bend your knees and position your feet, turn sideways and use the couch's arms as a backrest.
3. Place your front and back hands on your head.
4. Let your upper body lean over slightly, so your head can fall into your front hand, neck relaxed.
5. Apply the Mundo Method.

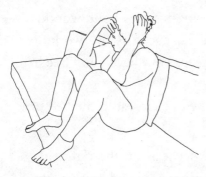

Fig. 19-5. Mundo Method, semi-reclining position

Lying-Down Position

To be honest, the lying-down position is my go-to because if I get a migraine it's usually a whopper from a surprise trigger ingredient ingested the day before — and the most I can do is lie in bed or on my couch and put my hands on my head. Sometimes I have to force myself to even begin the therapy, and sitting up doesn't feel like an option for me.

Follow this body positioning as written here because it's designed specifically to keep your back hand in very light contact with the back of your head. You *don't* want your back hand to be wedged between your head and a pillow because the weight of your head makes too much pressure on your palm. This creates a boomerang effect, and the headache can't release.

1. Lie down on a couch or bed, curled up in a semi-fetal position, with your head supported by a pillow, so it's level, not tilted up or down.
2. Lie on the *same side* that your headache is on — not completely on your side, but so you're situated halfway between your side and your back, on your shoulder blade.

   • You can place a pillow (or pillows) in front or in back (or both) of your body for stability.

- This three-quarter side position leaves your working arm free to move with your headache as you work on it with your thumb, and it keeps your back hand free to touch your head lightly.
- Your working arm will be the one closest to the bed or couch.
  - o That means, if your headache is on the right side, you'll be lying on your right side and working on your headache with your right thumb.
  - o And conversely, if your headache is on the left side, you'll be lying on your left side and working on your headache with your left thumb.

3. Rather than holding up the arm and elbow of your back hand, let them relax and flop over your head, so they make a little nest. For support you can also place a pillow under that arm, between it and your body or the bed.
4. If you need to change sides during a severe migraine, try rolling stomach side–down; it might be less jarring.

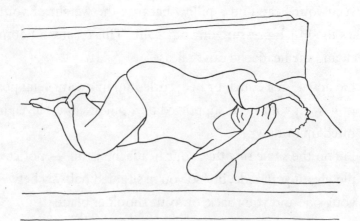

Fig. 19-6. **Mundo Method, lying-down position**

Practice Notes

I am happy to report that my clients and students learn how to reduce the frequency and intensity of their headaches and migraines so well that they don't have as many occasions to practice the Mundo Method. I hope this is happening for you right now as you integrate prevention practices into your daily life!

However, if you do get a headache, you now know how to use the innate tools at your fingertips to conquer it on the spot! And don't despair that you could be backsliding. Accidents and surprise triggers happen. Instead, reframe your pain as an opportunity to practice and get familiar with your headache's subtleties.

You can also balance your head with the Mundo Method even without an active headache or migraine. Actually, it's excellent to practice and get familiar with your head, use your hands in position, and work with sensations when you're not in pain or when your headache is very mild.

But please take note: Whenever you practice on yourself, whether with or without a headache, make sure to let the cycle complete according to the directions, so your head will be left in balance.

Recording Your Progress

When you get a headache or migraine — and after you've recovered — record an "HA" in your diary. Note the time it started, its intensity (on a pain scale of 1 to 10), your treatment — for instance the Mundo Method, any medication taken, self-massage, heat/cold — the treatment duration, and the time your headache ended. Keep it brief, something like: *9 AM HA #7, MM 1 hr, 12 PM better.*

Charting your acute therapy usage of the Mundo Method and self-massage will help you see your progress with hands-on treatments and your decreased reliance on pain-relief medications.

Part Five

The Deeper Realms
of Headache

20 Headaches, Somatic Shaping, and Trauma

My sincerest wish for you is that in the process of reading this book and implementing new practices, your headaches have decreased in frequency and intensity. If you have followed the program up to this point and are still searching for clues, you might need to look even more deeply to find out how and why you collect your stress or fall off your healthy habits wagon. Even though stress or diet can still play their roles, some headaches have underlying emotional causes as well.

In the preface, I described the process through which my long-standing chronic back pain was healed with an emotional release during breath work. After this happened, I became fascinated by the real-time intersection of pain, emotions, and the body, which also kept emerging in my clients' sessions. In the Always versus Never exercise, breathing sessions, meditation, and hands-on therapies, you have worked with your body, mind, and awareness in so many ways. You've learned to discover and release where and how you hold your stress, tension, and pain. Perhaps some roots of your pain, triggers, and patterns even rose to the surface and became exposed.

When people who have lived in pain are able to recognize, own, and release what has shaped them, they feel freed, as if a weight has been lifted off their shoulders. My client Carla's emotional hurt at five years old was reflected in her tight voice and inability to speak up for herself as an adult. In exploring her armoring, she noticed constriction in her throat, a collapse in her chest, and very shallow breathing. In facing the emotional hurt that resided in her voice and body, Carla released the underlying tension that had held her headaches in place — and started speaking up for herself.

In this chapter, we look at how and why somatic shaping gets created, and how this shaping can affect headaches.

What Shapes Us

Babies are open, sensitive, and full of wonder — they're the ultimate beginners. They live in a preverbal world where every sight, sound, touch, and mood is amplified. They feel everything that is around them because their filters haven't yet been set. In each moment they are learning about the world through the open channels of their senses, without thoughts, fears, and judgments getting in the way.

Although we enter the world as blank slates, we are shaped by our experiences — how we are touched, held, talked to, seen, loved, fed, cared for, and socialized — at least from the moment we are born (if not before). Our behavioral patterns are influenced by family, surroundings, society, and culture, from which we are always getting messages and signals. Even seemingly innocuous experiences can have a lasting impact.

As we receive and respond to experiences and messages, we embody what works for us and repeat it like a habit. As with riding a bike, once we've thoroughly learned, we do it without thinking. It becomes part of us.

Our somatic shaping is the structure we use to make the world coherent and loving for ourselves; it is a testament to our resilience. We adapt to and do whatever works in our environment to get love, feel safe, and survive, which then forms the construct of how we live in our bodies, think, feel, speak, act, listen, and see ourselves and the world.

The messages we get can literally shape us for a lifetime. For example, what shaping might result from messages like "Sit up straight," "Shut up," "Don't yell," "Don't tell," "Stop crying," and "Toughen up"? How would you be affected by labels like *great, beautiful, smart, wonderful, good,* and *cute*? What about *ugly, stupid, slow, retarded, silly,* or *bad*? Our core self — mind, body, emotions, and spirit — responds to all of this.[1]

Somatic Shaping and Headaches

Somatic shaping can be based on social as well as personal influences. Perhaps you copied how a favorite friend or relative smiled, laughed, stood, walked, talked, tilted her head, tossed her hair, tightened her jaw, or squinted her eyes. Maybe you wear tight jeans because they're in style, even though you can barely breathe. We adopt what we see in others because it's familiar, accepted, or admired.

Somatic shaping can occur over time and/or with one significant event. For example, if you are told once to stop crying, you might tighten your jaw and throat to choke back the tears. This behavior works, so you practice it again and again, and it becomes embodied, automatic. Or someone shames you about your weight, body, or bodily functions, and you learn to hold and contract parts of yourself. Or you are touched in an invasive, inappropriate way, so you tighten your body and shrink back into yourself in protection.

In these examples, the shaping is an instantaneous response, a choice deep down inside us that can be unconscious and imperceptible. When our choice of response restores us to a state of safety, comfort, and love, we continue to deploy it in similar situations. (Why not? It saved us!) This is how shaping can take place in the moment *and* over time.

Based on everything you've learned so far about the mind-body connection, can you see how these automatic behaviors, postures, facial expressions, and clothing choices might be connected to someone's headaches, or even your own?

Headaches and Trauma

Those original, delicious sensations of energy that once streamed through us as babies and children get squelched in somatic shaping around trauma and stress. We become tight, still, held, and numb, protecting or cut off from ourselves in any number of configurations, and this stagnation can be at the root of our pain. Thus, the source of pain is often beyond the purely physical.

Transformational somatic work that releases trauma is often a core part of reclaiming that part of yourself, healing pain, and moving beyond it. In this process, some clients share their trauma stories upfront. With others, the stories surface during the course of the work.

Whether you remember what originally happened or not, your shaping around trauma might still be influencing your present-day experiences and reactions. Perhaps a person, situation, or power dynamic is a conscious or unconscious reminder, so your survival brain kicks in and you check out, defer, or push back. Your body automatically goes with what it knows because it's how you've survived until now. Despite reality and your best efforts, you're powerless to respond to who or what is actually in front of you, and you again become that hurt child or rebellious teenager.

The unresolved emotional pain and yearning carried around in your body can be just as hurtful as scrapes and bruises — and often longer-lasting. This pain manifests in the way you hold your body, or ignore those tight shoulders and keep working, or take on too many responsibilities, or don't allow yourself to breathe and take a break — or always judge yourself, abdicate your best judgment, close yourself off from others, or push too hard. Whatever it is for you, ask yourself the *wonder vision* question, "How did I shape myself, perhaps to withstand a traumatic event or events, in a way that might be causing or underlying my pain now?"

Case Studies in Transforming Trauma and Pain

I feel honored to hold a safe space where clients can heal and tell their stories of pain and trauma. I have witnessed the melting away of barriers that keep them from their truest physical, mental, emotional, and spiritual selves. Going deeper somatically helped them understand and overcome their cycles of pain.

Here are some of their stories, with names and details changed.

Sophie

Sophie, who had a twenty-year history of migraine, did not remember her childhood sexual abuse until it emerged during her bodywork session. As a result of her trauma, she had unconsciously added excessive weight to her body, as if to provide a layer of protection. After facing her trauma, Sophie became empowered, took charge of her life, shed eighty pounds, and taught her husband how to relieve her migraines with the Mundo Method. She stopped going to the emergency room for shots of Demerol, previously her sole salvation.

Sophie later wrote: "I suffered from migraines for so long that I felt I was not in control. After a while, it breaks down your self-esteem and keeps you from so many things in life. I have since had the nerve to leave the job I was so unhappy with and start out in a new direction."

John

A programmer in his twenties, John was referred to me by his physician because he was now on disability. John had worked nonstop, coding at his computer. It's no wonder that he was unable to feel his neck and shoulders, or that his arms were going numb from overuse. When we first started working together, extremely light touch to his upper body, jaw, and chin felt painful to him. To get an idea of his sensitivity, barely touch the back of your forearm with your finger. That would have evoked an "ow."

Then John's story emerged: He had trained himself to ignore his pain in order to survive emotionally. When he was a teenager, his mother would mistreat him physically and deride him, saying things like "Shut your trap." What's worse, his mother subsequently had him institutionalized. John's feelings of betrayal were compounded at the facility when workers washed his mouth out with soap, just as his mother had done. The treatment he received was so invasive that he had to shut down access to his body, and to his very self. His jaw became perpetually locked and in pain, and he began to interpret any touch as danger.

We worked very slowly over time, using breathing and light touch work to soften the frozen numbness in his jaw, chin, face, head, shoulders, neck, and arms. As John became unfrozen and learned to trust that he wouldn't be hurt, his pain, tension, and migraines began to melt away. I also worked with him and his wife as a couple, helping them develop a language of touch that conveyed love, safety, and comfort.

Olivia

During Olivia's childhood, her parents often left her in the care of relatives, one of whom abused her sexually. She already felt abandoned by her parents, and then her abuser intimidated her into keeping the abuse a secret. She had trusted her family to protect her, but they betrayed her.

In her first months as my client, Olivia usually came to her session in the throes of a migraine. Her mood was off, her face pale, eyelids drooped. Her torso appeared turtle-shaped, with almost a dowager's hump in back, and her shoulders and head curved forward, making her chest collapse.

To the touch, her body and pain felt to me as if they were encased in an eggshell, so I would do extremely light, slow fascia easing. But the following day, her body would seize up, as if closing again in protection. Her body's held-down tension could not tolerate that much letting go and openness because it was so used to being "protected" (that is, closed down and shut off).

As Olivia released her emotional pain and reclaimed control of her body during breathing, bodywork, and coaching sessions, her shell began to soften. This eventually allowed her to do gentle exercise and core strengthening, which in turn increased her flexibility, energy, and stamina. She had already mastered the dietary, postural, breathing, and meditation practices, but this last piece of work helped her turn the corner on her migraines. Her mood and attitude slowly shifted from "victim of circumstance" to "woman of power," and her delightful sense of humor returned. The entire process took a year. After nearly fifty years of pain, Olivia was pain-free.

What Shaped You?

Becoming aware of *how* your body holds your history, including any trauma, can shed new light on your pain. What messages did you receive, and how did you shape in response — to get noticed, be invisible, or fit in? Whether positive or negative, conscious or unconscious, your early messages become embodied and can affect you long after the events occurred.

Did your migraines begin during a tumultuous time in your life, or after an accident or a traumatic event? Do you carry around your past in the form of bodily tension, loose boundaries, automatic reactions, or other coping mechanisms? As a child, how were you treated when you were sick or injured? Happy and healthy? When you spoke up or expressed yourself in various ways?

First It's an It...

When trying to shift ingrained patterns, even small changes are progress. At the same time, they can be difficult to maintain. If you're hard on yourself and expect instant change, remember, "Rome wasn't built in a day." As my fourth-grade teacher used to say, "First it's an *it*, then it's a *bit*, then it's a *habit*."

In that same way, your behaviors were built over time and have supported you in various ways. They've held your world together and kept it safe and coherent for a long time, so it makes sense that they still affect you, even as you envision and commit to change. To loosen their grip and reverse them takes working on yourself over time — at least one year, and even longer with a history of trauma. Body-centered therapies and practices that combine somatic awareness, breathing, bodywork, and movement can help you unwind unproductive patterns, create familiarity with sensations and feelings, and build new shaping that supports your vibrant well-being. Some clients also work with a psychotherapist in addition to somatic work.

Real change means more than stopping old habits. Get curious about what lies beneath those habits and how and why they were put into place. Then love yourself for trying and for all the work you have done so far and will continue to do.

If you have "aha" moments about connections between your somatic shaping and your headaches, add those revelations to your Headache Diary, even with just a word or two.

21 Embodied Wisdom: Your Feeling Self

We've been exploring what lies beneath bodily tension and holding, how people are shaped by their experiences, and how shaping can contribute to headaches. In this chapter, we shift focus away from activity toward inner states of feeling and being.

In making life changes, whether big or small, you are challenging your old shape and shedding what has been weighing you down. In doing so, you are also growing your capacity to be more present to your choices in each moment: to shop for and eat healthy foods, meditate, breathe, work on your tight neck and shoulders. And in the process, perhaps you are able to be more conscious and caring toward yourself and others when *executing* those choices. Mining your old habits for headache connections might have uncovered or brought more awareness to your emotions, feelings, and moods. Now what?

A common thread running through the practices of meditation, breathing, and touch is sensation. Using your touch, awareness, and mental focus, you have felt and worked with bodily, head, and headache sensations, such as pain, tightness, pulsations, knots, heat, and perhaps even a magnetic pull.

As you complete your headache healing journey, let's weave these threads together by revisiting the transformative body-centered work of somatics pioneers Drs. Gay and Kathlyn Hendricks and Dr. Richard Strozzi-Heckler, presented here in the form of an exercise and a practice. You will explore your emotional self through sensations and language and learn the practice of Centering as a way to come home to your body in each moment.

Feelings and Headaches

When you explore the emotional roots of your physical pain, you make the unconscious conscious. Emotions, even deeply buried emotions, live in the body. In the book *Molecules of Emotion*, Dr. Candace Pert details her groundbreaking scientific research, which shows how our emotions are carried by peptides that circulate throughout the body and fit like lock and key into our cells.[1] When you locate your feelings in your body and allow yourself to voice them, it creates more ease because you are facing and feeling what is true for you. Conversely, holding in your feelings, ignoring them, or feeling one way on the inside while acting differently on the outside creates tension in body and mind. Expressing without judgment, even to yourself, how you actually feel can bring a sense of relief and embodied peace.

Feeling Your Feelings: An Exercise

The honest simplicity of this sensitive, body-centered exercise, adapted from the work of Gay and Kathlyn Hendricks, can bring you face to face with what is true for you right now.[2] It's a vehicle for finding words and bodily locations for what has been unexpressed. You locate in your body each of your feelings (such as sadness, anger, fear, sexuality, guilt, shame, gratitude, and happiness), notice its sensations, and list what is true for you about that feeling until your list is complete. Then you repeat the process for the next feeling, and so on.

Lie comfortably on your back, arms by your sides, eyes closed.

First create a space of loving intention for yourself to hold throughout the process. Then softly speak aloud the following questions and your answers as you feel your body, your sensations, and your feelings. Go within and just feel. (The notes in parentheses are examples. There are no right or wrong answers.)

1. Where in your body do you feel sadness? Bring your awareness to feelings of sadness. ("I feel sadness in my throat, chest, and heart.")

2. What are the sensations connected to your feelings of sadness? (tightness, heaviness, a lump in my throat)

3. What do you feel sad about? Go with your "first thought, best thought" as you focus on the area in your body where you feel sadness.

4. Say softly, "I feel sad about _____" (or "I feel sad that _____") and let yourself feel it. Fill in the blank by saying whatever thought or memory comes up.

5. Repeat the phrase "I feel sad about _____," filling in the blank with whatever comes up next. Continue the process until you run out of things you feel sad about.

6. Return to step 1, and repeat the process for each feeling one by one, noticing what happens.

List of Feelings: I Feel...

- Sad
- Angry
- Afraid, fearful
- Sexual
- Guilty
- Ashamed
- Grateful
- Happy, joyful

How was that? Were some feelings or areas of your body more difficult to locate and feel than others? Did any thoughts, memories, or feelings emerge that you hadn't expected?

Being present to what you feel and where it lives in your body can relieve the emotional burden you have been carrying around. Perhaps the exercise has helped you realize something you need to do or change, something that's long overdue. If you truly honored your feelings, how might that impact your headaches? What things would you do differently if guided by your inner wisdom?

This quote from Gay and Kathlyn Hendricks's book *Conscious Loving: The Journey to Co-commitment* describes it beautifully:

> So often breakthroughs come right after people have let themselves feel and sense their emotions in their bodies. It is as if the universe has arranged it so that we cannot move forward before we let ourselves be where we are.[3]

Centering

The practice of Centering is a way to come home to your body and ground yourself on the earth, using your sensations to put yourself in balance. Centering shifts your awareness from your thinking to your feeling self and allows you to be fully present.

In his book *The Anatomy of Change*, Richard Strozzi-Heckler describes how being fully present — to sensations, attitudes, beliefs, behaviors, moods, and feelings — can help people understand and unwind the choices they have embodied over time. Centering is fundamental to this process.[4]

What Centering Is Good For

Since I first learned Centering from Richard in 1996 during professional somatics training (including its many adjunct forms and variations learned over the following ten years), one of the gifts this practice has given me — and by extension, my clients — is a different relationship with gravity. Instead of pulling up and away from or collapsing into gravity, I use it to balance my weight and presence.

I more readily feel it when I'm off-center, or triggered by a reaction, and then I recenter. The idea isn't that you are immune from being triggered, but that you know when you are, and, with practice, are able to shift in real time and recover more quickly. (I still get triggered, but my recovery time is more commonly minutes, hours, or days, instead of weeks and months!) Centering snaps me into the moment and keeps me from collecting internal tension. (And stacking my body, which is part of the practice, has also greatly helped my lower back.)

This practice lowers your center of gravity from your head to your body's gravitational center, your *hara* in Japanese (or *dan tien* in Chinese), a couple of inches below the navel. Focusing on center is also common to Eastern forms of martial arts and meditation. The practice is beneficial for headache sufferers, especially those who think and worry a lot. It helps manage stress, bodily tension, posture, and typical reactive patterns. Thus Centering opens the possibility of more choice, as well as positive outcomes, in situations in which you previously might have repeated old, unproductive stories or interactions.

When Do You Do It?

Centering is a dynamic, active practice that can be done anytime, anywhere. You can do it as part of a formal practice, whether alone or in a group, or you can center "in action," like when you're standing in line at the supermarket, riding the train, preparing to give a public talk, or engaging in conversation.

What Is It?

As described by Dr. Strozzi-Heckler, your center is more than a physical designation. It's symbolic too. Centering is a way to tune in to your body and align along the dimensions of length, width, and depth — each with its own physical and metaphorical distinctions.

Center is defined as being connected, present, and open…

- Connected — to your body (your self)
- Present — to others
- Open — to possibilities

…against the background of (or for the sake of) what you care about.

Most of us are used to focusing on one of these — we're connected, present, *or* open — but not all of them at once. For example, you might be connected to your body but not present to the person in front of you (like at the gym). Or perhaps you're paying attention to someone you are talking with but not connected to your own body. Or you're connected and present but closed to possibilities — or maybe not invested in what you're doing. Being centered is holding everything in balance.

Centering, Meet Armoring!

Armoring is another somatics term for our shaping and how we contract parts of ourselves in order to survive, feel safe, fit in, and get love. Dr. Wilhelm Reich, a contemporary of Freud's, coined the term *character armoring* to describe the embodied demeanors and behavioral traits that keep us from our natural, energetic aliveness, creativity, and expression. Armoring is like an inner and outer shield that we mold in any number of ways. We shape-shift, squeeze tight, or vacate parts of our bodies to become small or tall, attractive or unattractive, invisible or flamboyant, smart or dumb, tough or a pushover…you name it. From within that shape, however, it can be difficult to act differently or see the world in another light.

According to Chinese medicine and other healing modalities, energy flows lengthwise through the body. When we armor ourselves, we tighten and contract in protection, which constricts the flow of energy and cuts us off from feelings and sensations. It's like pinching a water hose or a balloon and stemming the flow of water or air.

In Centering, you use your awareness to walk through cross sections of your body, called *armoring bands*, and let go of any habitual holding in each area. If you find an area that seems to be perpetually tight or sore, with this practice you can help retrain your body by making the unconscious conscious. By restoring flow throughout your body, you can begin to unwind your pain and feel more alive.

Dimensions of Center

The three dimensions of Center are length, width, and depth, and each is physical and relational.

Length is the vertical line of the body — our higher consciousness and earthly nature.

As humans, we are the vertical animal; we walk on two legs, not four. We're conscious: we know that we know. When the body is centered in length, it is stacked vertically, and we are balanced from top to bottom. We soar to the heavens while being grounded on the earth, part of the web of life.

When we're off-center in length, there's a distortion in that balance. You know how it feels when you're sick or feeling the weight of the world: you feel pulled down by gravity, collapsed. Conversely, do you know people who seem so ungrounded, they're like hummingbirds that can't alight?

Width is the body side to side — and our social space.

When the body is centered in width, it is balanced right to left, with weight equally distributed on both feet. Width is the social space — you in relation to the world. You're not just forward-facing; you and your energy extend 360 degrees around your body. Your field doesn't end at your skin border — it extends beyond your body. While you're facing what you are doing, your peripheral vision is open.

When we're off-center in width, there's a distortion in that balance: weight unequally distributed left to right; torqued or turning away; half out the door. It's like a person at a party who is just about to leave a conversation — partially turned away and ready to move on. Instead of being open, we get tunnel vision, and our peripheral vision narrows or closes.

Depth is the body front to back — and our history.

You move forward through the world, with the future in front of you; your past is behind you, at your back. You change and grow, yet you carry your history with you.

When we're off-center in depth, there's a distortion in that balance: It can be hard to let people in. Maybe you know someone who holds his cards close, and closes himself off from his history. Imbalance in depth might show up as a person who is unable to reveal deep emotions, and it might explain why some people can't keep a secret and tend to spill the beans.

Centering Practice

Bringing it all together, let's center!

SETUP

- Stand, or if that's not possible, sit or lie on your back with your legs extended.
- Rest your tongue on the roof of your mouth, letting your

teeth slightly part. Place your feet parallel on the floor, hip-distance apart, knees soft. Your body is stacked — ears, shoulders, hips, knees, and feet aligned vertically. Place your arms by your sides.

- Notice your sensations throughout the practice as you follow along and walk your awareness through your body.
- Let go of any holding you might feel.
- During the process, you might feel a sense of flow, tingling, pulsation, vibration, temperature, heat, or cold. You might sense your body in gravity (heavy, light, held, loose, open, closed); you might experience qualities of objects (sheet-metal plate, board, cord); and moods, thoughts, feelings, and memories might come to the surface.

CENTER IN LENGTH

Here you are Centering your body top to bottom — and above and below you. Walk your awareness through your armoring bands, the cross sections of your body, all the way around and through.

- Read the list, then close your eyes, and name each area in your mind as you walk through it.
- Bring your awareness to each band, be fully present to it and to any sensations, then soften around any holding.
- Starting at the top of your head, bring your mind to each band in the following order:
  o Forehead, eyes (including the eye sockets and around the back of the head, like wraparound shades)
  o Jaw, jawline, chin
  o Neck: front, sides, back; inside, your throat and voice
  o Shoulder girdle: shoulder ridge, upper chest, upper arms, upper back; inside, the area around your heart
  o Ribs, diaphragm, mid-back

- o Belly, solar plexus, lower back
- o Drop your breathing into your lower abdomen. Place your palm over your center, an inch or two below your belly button, and feel your hand pushed out by your breath on the inhale and move closer to your spine on the exhale.
- o Lower abdomen, pelvic girdle, sacrum, buttocks
- o Sphincters, genital and anal (squeeze and release them a few times to let go of any holding)
- o Thighs, knees, legs, ankles, feet, soles of feet

As you feel the weight of your body in gravity, honor your connection to heaven and earth, life and all its living creatures, your grounding with the earth, and your aspirations in life.

Now, reverse your direction. Starting at the soles of your feet, bring your awareness up through each armoring band and notice if anything has changed from your first pass. When you get back to the top of your head, complete Centering in length by slowly opening your eyes and letting "the world come to you."

CENTER IN WIDTH

This is your body side to side — and your social space. Keeping your eyes open, feel yourself extend into the world 360 degrees around.

- Notice the balance of your weight between left and right and side to side. Notice whether one side is torqued forward or turned away.
- Come into balance.
- Rotate your arms, so your palms are open, facing forward. Extend your fingers, and open yourself to the world.
- Soften your gaze, and open your peripheral vision to see to the front and sides.

CENTER IN DEPTH

Now Center your body front to back — your history and future.

- Close your eyes and feel your body front to back.
- Notice how you face your future and carry your history behind you, in your back.
- As you move forward in the world, feel your back.

WHAT DO YOU NOTICE?

Notice how you feel and whether anything is different. Do you feel calmer, less stressed, more accepting of what is? Are you ready to ask for what you need or want? What's your mood? Did thoughts, memories, or feelings arise when you took time to just be and feel within yourself while also being open to the world? Were some dimensions and areas of your body and self more accessible than others? How about more or less comfortable?

Try taking your centered self out for a spin. Staying present to your body, begin to walk around. Notice the room or area and what's in it, including people and animals. Do things feel or look different when you are centered? What do you imagine would change about the way you engage, interact, and connect with life if you were centered more often? How might it affect your headaches?

Finding Peace

I hope this program has provided you with a positive, transformative journey — and continues to do so going forward.

I'm imagining a new life for you where you continue to nourish and take care of yourself on all levels. A life where you keep breathing into discovery, forgiving yourself and others, and releasing fear and anxiety. Gather around you the support, love, peace, and strength that you need, starting from within yourself. You are magnificently resilient and have done a great job! Now let's complete.

Conclusion:
Embodying Your New Life

*I*t's time for congratulations! Bravo! You've done an amazing job. What an achievement it is to take your headaches, literally, into your own hands.

And now, after all your dedication to lifestyle changes, somatic practices, self-care therapies, and inner work, you have come to the end of your headache journey. You are entering a new future in a life without headaches and full of possibilities, one you have worked hard on and prepared for. You have the tools, and you're ready. This is your commencement!

To complete the program, let's recognize, evaluate, appreciate, and honor your successes and progress. You will assess your current state by filling out the Mundo Program Self-Evaluation and comparing your new answers to those in the Headache History Questionnaire from chapter 3.

Claim and Appreciate Your Success!

Claiming and appreciating your success is an important part of the headache healing process. It helps to remember where you began and realize how far you have come.

By appreciating your enormous accomplishment in healing your own headaches with mind-body self-care, you can feel the impact of your commitments and actions, leave behind your painful chapters, and move on with your life. The more you can fully own how far you have come and really let that sink in, the more you will remember how you got here and where to look if you lose your way.

Let's look at all you have accomplished. Through somatic self-care, as an active reader of *The Headache Healer's Handbook*, you have:

- learned ways to assert your power to heal yourself rather than suffer,
- gained expertise in recognizing and managing a variety of headache triggers,
- developed a somatic sensibility to see, feel, and work with your body and self,
- learned how to relax your tension and holding and prevent your headaches through breathing, meditation, gentle exercise, and self-massage,
- used specialized touch and focused concentration to relieve a headache or migraine on the spot,
- explored the deeper emotional connections to your pain and health, and
- triumphed over your pain and moved beyond it.

May I just say "That's amazing!" By working with yourself in this way and expanding your awareness of your attitudes, moods, beliefs, and behaviors, you have embodied the strength to direct your destiny.

Mundo Program Self-Evaluation

Reflect on how you are feeling and answer the questions. Circle, highlight, or write in your answers.

1. Date: _____

2. Name: _____

3. How often do you get headaches now?

   # per week: _____ *or* # per month: _____ *or* # per year: _____

4. How long do your headaches usually last now?

   # of minutes: _____ *or* # of hours: _____ *or* # of days: _____

5. Indicate the usual intensity of your headaches by circling a number on the pain scale.

   0　　1　　2　　3　　4　　5　　6　　7　　8　　9　　10
   |　　　　　　　　　　　　　　　　　　　　　　　　　　　　|
   No pain　　　　　　　　　　　　　　　　　　　　　　Most intense
   　　　　　　　　　　　　　　　　　　　　　　　　　pain imaginable

6. Do you use self-massage for headache relief and prevention?

   Always　　　Often　　　Sometimes　　　Rarely　　　Never

7. Does it work?

   Always　　　Often　　　Sometimes　　　Rarely　　　Never

8. Do you use Mundo Method hands-on therapy for headache relief?

   Always　　　Often　　　Sometimes　　　Rarely　　　Never

9. Does it work?

   Always　　　Often　　　Sometimes　　　Rarely　　　Never

10. How long does it take for the Mundo Method to work?

    # of minutes: _____ *or* # of hours: _____

11. How often, in total, do you do stress reduction practices, such as meditation, breathing, Centering, and desk exercises?

    7 days/wk　　5–6 days/wk　　3–4 days/wk　　1–2 days/wk　　0 days/wk

12. Do the above stress reduction practices help your headaches?
    ❏ Yes   ❏ No   ❏ Maybe
    If yes, which practices? Please describe how they help: _____

    _____

13. Do the above practices improve your daily life?
    ❏ Yes   ❏ No   ❏ Maybe
    If yes, describe how: _____

14. How often do you exercise?

    7 days/wk   5–6 days/wk   3–4 days/wk   1–2 days/wk   0 days/wk
    Describe what you do and for how long: _____

    _____

15. Have you changed any of the following lifestyle factors during the
    program? If so, does it help your headaches? (Circle your answers.)

LIFESTYLE FACTOR	CHANGED?		DOES IT HELP?		
Nutrition (foods)	Yes	No	Yes	No	Maybe
Eating habits (times and/or frequency)	Yes	No	Yes	No	Maybe
Water intake	Yes	No	Yes	No	Maybe
Caffeine intake	Yes	No	Yes	No	Maybe
Alcohol intake	Yes	No	Yes	No	Maybe
Exercise habits	Yes	No	Yes	No	Maybe
Attention to feelings	Yes	No	Yes	No	Maybe
Awareness of body	Yes	No	Yes	No	Maybe
Other: _____	Yes	No	Yes	No	Maybe

16. Have you reduced your medication intake since beginning this pro-
    gram?   ❏ Yes   ❏ No
    If yes, describe: _____

    _____

17. If you are currently taking any medications (including OTC), for headaches or for anything else, please indicate below, including details about dosage, frequency, and effectiveness.

Medication	Dosage/Amount	How often?	Helps headache?	
_____	_____	_____	❏ Yes	❏ No
_____	_____	_____	❏ Yes	❏ No
_____	_____	_____	❏ Yes	❏ No
_____	_____	_____	❏ Yes	❏ No

18. Of everything you have done to heal your headaches, what has made the biggest difference?

19. What did you used to do, before you started following the Mundo Program?

20. Rate how you feel upon completion of the program.

    Excellent Much better Better Same Worse Much worse

21. Add anything else you'd like to include:

Before and After

Read over your self-evaluation. Then reflect back to how you felt before you began the Mundo Program: how many headaches you had and how often; how sick you felt; how much your pain affected your outlook, energy, and mood — and your family, school, work, and social life.

Then turn back to the Headache History Questionnaire that you completed in chapter 3 and read it over. Do you remember that person? Look at your whole picture as you take stock of where you began and how far you have come.

What is different? What has changed in your body, mind, emotions, and spirit? How is that change reflected in your life, and how will you sustain the changes over time? What commitments can you make and what kind of support systems can you build to help you stay on track?

Keeping Up with the Changes

It's almost universal that when we start feeling better, we're able to increase our activity levels and live at a faster pace. And why shouldn't we? We are finally beginning to feel normal. It's fantastic!

But then we get so, so busy that we run out of time to do the practices that made us feel better in the first place. Our healthy routines start falling away, bit by bit, as we have less time to shop for healthy foods, eat regular meals, drink enough water, work out, breathe, meditate, and do self-massage. To keep up with our increased activity load, we might add an afternoon tea or café latte, which can also disrupt our sleep. Then, "out of the blue," we're getting more headaches again.

It happens. It's life, and we're only human.

Stay True to Your Path

Headache healing is not magic, and you didn't arrive here by accident. You walked the path step by step, so you know the journey. You are self-maintaining, and you no longer need your Headache Diary to stay on track.

If you get off track, you know what to do: take an inventory of all the exercises, attitudes, and practices that brought you to wellness. If you have dropped or cut back on some of these, return to any related chapters in the book to refresh your memory. You can resume your Headache Diary for a month or so; you might discover patterns or realize you have let slide certain activities or practices that have helped you before.

Whatever it is — breathing, meditation, self-massage, protein, frequent meals and snacks, water — add it back into your routine, and see what happens. As always, your diary can be your readout, showing the results of any changes you make — and you'll have a record. Once you are solidly back on track, you can let go of it again.

Life Minus Headaches

Now that you are a *former* headache sufferer, it's time to move beyond living with pain as your defining narrative and into a revised future. So much of your prior life was centered around pain; what is it like to live without it?

Open the door to a life without pain. How do you want to live now? What will fulfill you? What will you contribute as a unique being during your time on the planet?

If you have curbed your social and family activities, you might devote some time to consciously re-creating yourself. If you have been accustomed to being sick and tired, now's the time to restore pleasure and enjoyment, without fear that the other shoe will drop. What have you always wanted to do, if not for your headaches and migraines? The art is to create a balanced life where you can enjoy yourself while maintaining good practices that will keep you from the old patterns. You can expand into new dimensions of passion and creativity that as a chronic migraine sufferer you couldn't have imagined.

Be proudly defiant! Having headaches and migraines is not the foregone conclusion or your life sentence: it is within your reach to live a headache-free life. And you have fulfilled that goal. What's next?

Envision the headache-free life you would like to create. Let your path be revealed as you keep trueing your whole self — mind, body emotions, and spirit — to your path, like an adventurer navigates by the North Star. Affirm it. Write it. Paint it. Speak it. Sing it.

Whatever it is, my deepest hope and prayer is that this new life brings you joy, pleasure, excitement, and fulfillment. Whether it keeps you up at night out of sheer joy or lets you sleep deeply and restoratively, let this life be beyond the world of pain and suffering. May your headaches be a faded memory, and may you blossom into and embody your true self and walk steadily on your path.

Acknowledgments

"The road is long with many a winding turn
that leads us to who knows where, who knows where."
— **Bob Russell and Bobby Scott**

*E*xploration and discovery are at the heart of this book and my path of following countless trails prompted by curiosity. Throughout my life I have been blessed with brilliant teachers (many of whom no longer grace this world) — guides, mentors, clients, colleagues, friends, and family — who believed in me, heard me, trusted my work, and entertained my unconventional theories and questions about everything. Some conversations have lasted for years, while others were only a sentence, perhaps a chance meeting. For all this and more, I am forever grateful.

My savvy agent, Susan Lee Cohen, luckily said yes and guided me to the perfect publishing home for this book. Editor Alice Peck had graciously referred me to Susan after reading my proposal.

The tireless team at New World Library brought *The Headache Healer's Handbook* to life: Executive Editor Jason Gardner, my editor, was excited about the book, heard my voice and meaning right away, and patiently and generously supported me throughout the publishing process. Managing Editor Kristen Cashman kept the production ship on course and prompted me to polish any remaining cloudy stones. Assistant Editor Joel Prins coordinated the endorsements and performed final editorial checks. Art Director Tracy Cunningham deftly prepared my illustrations for publication and conveyed a mood of peaceful healing with her cover design. Tona Pearce Myers designed and typeset an interior that headache sufferers can read with ease. Copyeditor Patricia Heinicke and proofreader Tanya Fox helped me clarify my language to express what I really meant. The buzzing hive of New World Library's marketing department — Publicity Director Monique Muhlenkamp, Marketing Director Munro Magruder, and Senior Publicist Kim Corbin — is ramping up as we go to press. Freelance photographer extraordinaire Claire Holt took my headshot for the back cover and made me feel camera comfy.

My illustration models — Julia Halpin, Jaime Shannon, David Berman, Nadine Mundo, and Elaine Collins — kindly provided the poses I needed to bring my written instructions to life. My daughters, Rena Croshere and Nadine Mundo, insisted, "Mom, you do the illustrations," despite my initial doubts. Artist Mark Schlichting described a low-tech path to my creating them, and it worked.

Over the years my generous writing and publishing teachers, mentors, and colleagues have offered invaluable lessons and insights: My writing teacher, Rowland Barber, said, "to write is to seek the truth," and taught me to "first write, and then rewrite, rewrite, rewrite...." He delivered enthusiastic critiques typed on stationery, and I wish he were here to read my debut work. I'm indebted to the sage publishing and writing advice of Ken Sherman, William Meyers, and Nancy Shanteau, my whiz Somatic Coach; my former editors, Laura Bonazzoli and Naomi Lucks; Hay House Online Writer's Workshop; and The Binders openhearted writing community.

Innumerable medical, health, wellness, and research profession-als in the fields of headache, pain, neurology, nutrition, and health education acknowledged and facilitated my work at each juncture: David Bresler, PhD, LAc, advised me to "get a license to touch." At UCLA, Susan L. Perlman, MD, referred my first clients; Jeffrey Gornbein, DPH, put me on the research train; John C. Liebeskind, PhD, and Joseph Janeti, PhD, discussed pain and the mind-body connection. Lee Kudrow, Sr., MD, encouraged my work after his impromptu Mundo Method treatment at a patio table. Richard L. Shames, MD, gave me my first physician testimonial when I "stopped his headache on the spot." Joyce Selkow, MS, RDN, ad-vised me on nutrition, health, and business; Gina Gallitero, MPH, hired me at Kaiser Permanente; and Otilia M. Tiutin, DNM, PhD, hired me at Hill Physicians Medical Group. Richard B. Lipton, MD, accepted our team's headache research study for peer-reviewed jour-nal publication and conference poster session. Alexander Mauskop, MD, referred patients to my practice and classes in New York City; I'm honored to have the knowledgeable, holistic perspective of this esteemed medical professional enrich the pages of the book's foreword.

My exceptional energy-work, healing, and somatics teachers changed my life, and their lessons invigorate me and inform my awareness every day. Healing teacher Kate McGovern and qigong master Joe Lopez taught me how to run energy through the body; Roger Hirsh, LAc, understood about drawing energy from plants to ease my carpal tunnel symptoms and referred me to Joe. Creator of Therapeutic Touch Dora Kunz told me, "Oh, you must breathe," when giving a treatment. Thelma Moss, PhD, and John Hubacher, MA, who had conducted biofield research at UCLA Parapsychology Lab, let me pick their brains; John suggested a breathing workshop with Mitchell May, PhD, who opened the door to transformative breathing and the Hendrickses. Gay Hendricks, PhD, Kathlyn Hendricks, PhD, Richard Strozzi-Heckler, PhD, and Staci Haines, MA, showed me the healing power of somatic transformation and introduced me to the unity of sensation, movement, breathing, feelings, moods, language, actions, and touch.

The love and support of my family and friends mean everything. My mom, late dad, brother, children, grandchildren, aunts, uncles, and cousins; my dear, beloved extended family of friends from The Farm in Tennessee and from California, New York, and beyond who have been there for me, prayed for my success, and encouraged my journey through many peaks and valleys: thank you — my world would be empty without you!

Endnotes

Preface

1. Richard B. Lipton, Walter F. Stewart, Seymour Diamond, Merle L. Diamond, and Michael L. Reed, "Prevalence and Burden of Migraine in the United States: Data from the American Migraine Study II," *Headache* 41, no. 7 (July 12, 2001): 646–57; Walter F. Stewart, Richard B. Lipton, David D. Celentano, and Michael L. Reed, "Prevalence of Migraine Headache in the United States: Relation to Age, Income, Race, and Other Sociodemographic Factors," *JAMA* 267, no. 1 (January 1, 1992): 64–69.
2. Paul E. Stang and Jane T. Osterhaus, "Impact of Migraine in the United States: Data from the National Health Interview Survey," *Headache* 33, no. 1 (January 1993): 29–35.
3. Teresa Wilson, Kelly Keller, Fawn McCloud, Jan Mundo, and Carla A. Lee, "The Cost-Effectiveness of a Prophylactic Migraine Programme as Contrasted to Pharmacological Migraine Treatment," *Cephalalgia: International Journal of Headache* 21, no. 4 (May 2001): 368.

Chapter 1. Putting Relief in Your Hands

1. "Migraine Facts," Migraine Research Foundation (website), December 3, 2017, http://migraineresearchfoundation.org/about-migraine/migraine-facts.
2. Susan Hutchinson, *The Woman's Guide to Managing Migraine: Understanding the Hormone Connection to Find Hope and Wellness* (New York: Oxford University Press, 2013), 7.

3. X. H. Hu, L. E. Markson, R. B. Lipton, W. F. Stewart, and M. L. Berger, "Burden of Migraine in the United States: Disability and Economic Costs," *Archives of Internal Medicine* 159, no. 8 (April 26, 1999): 813–18.

4. Scott W. Powers et al., "The Childhood and Adolescent Migraine Prevention (CHAMP) Study: A Report on Baseline Characteristics of Participants," *Headache* (2016), doi:10.1111/head.12810.

5. "International Classification of Headache Disorders," 3rd ed. (ICHD-3), beta version, International Headache Society, 2013, section 1, "Migraine," https://www.ichd-3.org/1-migraine, and section 2, "Tension-Type Headache," https://my.clevelandclinic.org/health/diseases/6170-headaches-rebound-headaches.

Chapter 2. What's Your Headache Type?

1. "International Classification of Headache Disorders," 3rd ed. (ICHD-3), beta version, International Headache Society, 2013, https://www.ichd-3.org.

2. Nicola J. Giffin, Richard B. Lipton, Stephen D. Silberstein, J. Oleson, and P. J. Goadsby, "The Migraine Postdrome: An Electronic Diary Study," *Neurology* 87, no. 3 (June 2016): 309–13.

3. Susan Hutchinson, *The Woman's Guide to Managing Migraine: Understanding the Hormone Connection to find Hope and Wellness* (New York: Oxford University Press, 2013), 9.

4. Lee Kudrow, "Response of Cluster Headache Attacks to Oxygen Inhalation," *Headache: The Journal of Head and Face Pain* 21, no. 1 (1981): 1–4.

Chapter 4. The Mind-Body-Headache Connection

1. Eleanor Criswell, *Biofeedback and Somatics: Toward Personal Evolution* (Novato, CA: Freeperson Press, 1995), 40.

2. Marvin Karlins and Lewis M. Andrews, *Biofeedback: Turning On the Power of Your Mind* (New York: Lippincott Williams & Wilkins, 1972), 74.

3. Joseph D. Sargent, Elmer E. Green, and E. Dale Walters, "The Use of Autogenic Feedback Training in a Pilot Study of Migraine and Tension Headaches," *Headache: The Journal of Head and Face Pain* 12, no. 3 (1972): 120–24.

4. Jose L. Medina, Seymour Diamond, and Mary A. Franklin, "Biofeedback Therapy for Migraine," *Headache: The Journal of Head and Face Pain* 16, no. 3 (1976): 115–18.

5. Alan C. Turin and William G. Johnson, "Biofeedback Therapy for Migraine Headaches," *Archives of General Psychiatry* 33, no. 4 (1976): 517–19.

6. Joseph D. Sargent, Patricia Solbach, Lolafaye Coyne, Herbert Spohn, and John Segerson, "Results of a Controlled, Experimental, Outcome Study of

Nondrug Treatments for the Control of Migraine Headaches," *Journal of Behavioral Medicine* 9, no. 3 (1986): 291–323.

7. Kenneth R. Mitchell and Daphne M. Mitchell, "Migraine: An Exploratory Treatment Application of Programmed Behavior Therapy Techniques," *Journal of Psychosomatic Research* 15, no. 2 (1971): 137–57.

8. Criswell, *Biofeedback and Somatics*, 14.

9. Clyde W. Ford, "Healing the Body Personal, Healing the Body Politic" (workshop, Sixth International Somatics Congress: The Living Body, San Francisco, CA, October 18–22, 1995).

10. Gay Hendricks and Kathlyn Hendricks, "Survival Vision and Wonder Vision" (training presentation, Conscious Relationship Transformation Professional Certification Program, The Hendricks Institute, Tiburon, CA, 1994).

11. Shunryu Suzuki, *Zen Mind, Beginner's Mind: Informal Talks on Zen Meditation and Practice* (New York and Tokyo: Weatherhill, 1970), 21.

12. Ted Kaptchuk and Franklin Miller, "Placebo Effects in Medicine," *New England Journal of Medicine* 373, no. 1 (July 2, 2015): 8–9.

13. Benika Pinch, "More Than Just a Sugar Pill: Why the Placebo Effect Is Real," Science in the News (SITN), Harvard Graduate School of the Arts and Sciences (website), September 14, 2016, http://sitn.hms.harvard.edu/flash/2016 /just-sugar-pill-placebo-effect-real.

14. Slavenka Kam-Hansen, Moshe Jakubowski, John M. Kelley, Irving Kirsch, David C. Hoaglin, Ted Kaptchuk, and Rami Burstein, "Altered Placebo and Drug Labeling Changes the Outcome of Episodic Migraine Attacks," *Science Translational Medicine* 6, no. 218 (January 8, 2014): 218ra5.

15. Ted Kaptchuk, Elizabeth Friedlander, John Kelley, M. Norma Sanchez, Efi Kokkotou, Joyce Singer, Magda Kowalczykowski, Franklin Miller, Irving Kirsch, and Anthony Lembo, "Placebos without Deception: A Randomized Controlled Trial in Irritable Bowel Syndrome," *PLOS One* 5, no. 12 (December 22, 2010): e15591.

Chapter 5. The Chinese Menu Theory

1. The American Council on Headache Education with Lynne M. Constantine and Suzanne Scott, "Potential Migraine Triggers," in *Migraine: The Complete Guide* (New York: Dell, 1994), 60.

Chapter 6. Dietary Triggers

1. "Caffeine Content of Popular Drinks," University of Utah, College of Science, Department of Mathematics (website), https://www.math.utah

.edu/~yplee/fun/caffeine.html; "Caffeine and Headaches," Cleveland Clinic (website), December 29, 2014, https://my.clevelandclinic.org/health/articles /caffeine-and-headache.

2. "Low-Tyramine Diet for Migraine," National Headache Foundation (website), October 25, 2007, https://www.headaches.org/2007/10/25/low -tyramine-diet-for-migraine.

Chapter 7. Environmental, Lifestyle, and Physical Triggers

1. Russel Davis, "Eco-Friendly LED Light Bulbs Found to Cause Increase in Headaches," Natural News (website), August 3, 2017, https://www.natural news.com/2017-08-03-eco-friendly-led-light-bulbs-found-to-cause -increase-in-headaches.html.

2. Anna Gryglas, "Allergic Rhinitis and Chronic Daily Headaches: Is There a Link?" *Current Neurology and Neuroscience Reports* 16 (2016): 33; and "Allergic Rhinitis, Sinusitis, and Rhinosinusitis," American Academy of Otolaryngology — Head and Neck Surgery (website), accessed February 6, 2018, http://www.entnet.org/content/allergic-rhinitis-sinusitis-and-rhinosinusitis.

Chapter 8. Medication and Hormonal Triggers

1. "International Classification of Headache Disorders," 3rd ed. (ICHD-3), beta version, International Headache Society, 2013, https://www.ichd-3 .org/8-headache-attributed-to-a-substance-or-its-withdrawal/8-2 -medication-overuse-headache-moh.

2. Hans-Christoph Diener and Zaza Katsarava, "Medication Overuse Headache," *Current Medical Research and Opinion* 17, suppl. 1 (2001), http://www .medscape.com/viewarticle/429667_4.

3. ICHD-3 beta, https://www.ichd-3.org/8-headache-attributed-to-a-substance -or-its-withdrawal/8-2-medication-overuse-headache-moh.

4. Susan Hutchinson, *The Woman's Guide to Managing Migraine: Understanding the Hormone Connection to find Hope and Wellness* (New York: Oxford University Press, 2013), 81.

5. "Rebound Headaches: Causes," Mayo Clinic (website), accessed October 21, 2017, https://www.mayoclinic.org/diseases-conditions/rebound-headaches /symptoms-causes/syc-20377083; "Headaches: Rebound Headaches," Cleveland Clinic (website), accessed March 16, 2018, https://my.clevelandclinic .org/health/diseases/6170-headaches-rebound-headaches; Espen Saxhaug Kristoffersen and Christofer Lundqvist, "Medication-Overuse Headache: Epidemiology, Diagnosis and Treatment," *Therapeutic Advances in Drug*

Safety 5, no. 2 (2014): 87–99; and Hutchinson, *The Woman's Guide to Managing Migraine*, 63.

6. Alexander Mauskop and Barry Fox, *What Your Doctor May Not Tell You about Migraines: The Breakthrough Program That Can Help End Your Pain*, (New York: Warner Books, 2001), 86.

7. Stewart J. Tepper, "Spotlight On: Neuromodulation Devices for Headache," American Migraine Foundation (website), May 25, 2017, https://american migrainefoundation.org/understanding-migraine/spotlight-neuromodulation -devices-headache.

8. Hutchinson, *The Woman's Guide to Managing Migraine*, 7; and Simona Sacco et al., "Migraine in Women: The Role of Hormones and Their Impact on Vascular Diseases," *The Journal of Headache and Pain* 13, no. 3 (2012): 177–89, https://www.ncbi.nlm.nih.gov/pmc/articles/PMC3311830.

9. Hutchinson, *The Woman's Guide to Managing Migraine*, 22.

10. Ibid., 132.

11. Ibid., 9.

12. Ibid., 116.

13. Ibid., 118.

14. Ibid., 43; and Richard B. Lipton, C. Mark Sollars, and Dawn C. Buse, "Epidemiology, Progression, Prognosis, and Comorbidity of Migraine," in *Neurology in Practice Series: Headache* (West Sussex, UK: Wiley-Blackwell, 2013), 70.

Chapter 9. Diet for Migraine Prevention

1. Rodolfo Low, *Victory over Migraine: The Breakthrough Study That Explains What Causes It and How It Can Be Completely Prevented through Diet* (New York: Henry Holt, 1987), 51.

2. R. K. Johnson, L. J. Appel, M. Brands, B. V. Howard, M. Lefevre, R. H. Lustig, F. Sacks, L. M. Steffen, and J. Wylie-Rosett, on behalf of the American Heart Association Nutrition Committee of the Council on Nutrition, Physical Activity, and Metabolism and the Council on Epidemiology and Prevention, "Dietary Sugars Intake and Cardiovascular Health: A Scientific Statement from the American Heart Association," *Circulation*, vol. 120 (2009): 1011–20.

3. Louise Hagler, ed., *The Farm Vegetarian Cookbook, Revised Edition* (Summertown, TN: Book Publishing Company, 1978), 58.

4. Ibid., 12.

5. Johnson et al., "Dietary Sugars Intake and Cardiovascular Health."

6. "Dr. Weil's Anti-Inflammatory Diet," Dr. Weil (website), https://www

.drweil.com/health-wellness/health-centers/aging-gracefully/dr-weils-anti
-inflammatory-diet.

Chapter 11. Breathing In, Breathing Out

1. Thích Nhất Hanh, *Touching Peace: Practicing the Art of Mindful Living* (Berkeley, CA: Parallax Press, 1992), 13.
2. For their presentation of these exercises, see "Centered Breathing" in Gay Hendricks and Kathlyn Hendricks, *At the Speed of Life: A New Approach to Personal Change through Body-Centered Therapy* (New York: Bantam, 1993), 180.
3. Mitchell May, breathing workshop, California, circa 1992.
4. Hendricks and Hendricks, *At the Speed of Life*, 183.

Chapter 12. Being Still: Mindfulness and Headaches

1. Thích Nhất Hanh, *Touching Peace: Practicing the Art of Mindful Living* (Berkeley, CA: Parallax Press, 1992), 13.
2. Sylvia Boorstein, "When the Going Gets Tough, the Tough…Meditate: Spiritual Practices to Calm the Mind and Support the Heart during Difficult Times" lecture, with Sylvia Boorstein and David Ingber, Sparks: Live Conversation Series, New York, June 1, 2016, romemu.org.

Chapter 14. The Zen of Exercise and Headaches

1. I've learned these exercises from various places over the years — some as a child (from eye doctors), some as a pregnant woman and when doing qigong, some from gym class warm-ups as a teen and adult. I rediscovered some of them in the following book: Harry C. Ehrmantraut, *Headaches: The Drugless Way to Lasting Relief!* (Berkeley, CA: Celestial Arts, 1987), 54. He called his exercises "Face and Scalp Calisthenics" and "Neck and Shoulder Rejuvenators."

Chapter 20. Headaches, Somatic Shaping, and Trauma

1. I learned about somatic shaping, trauma, and resilience in professional training courses with Staci K. Haines, MA, and Denise Benson, MFT ("Somatics and Trauma I," San Francisco, CA, 2002) and with Richard

Strozzi-Heckler, PhD (Somatic Coaching Program, Petaluma, CA, 1996–2005).

Chapter 21. Embodied Wisdom: Your Feeling Self

1. Candace Pert, *Molecules of Emotion: Why You Feel the Way You Feel* (New York: Scribner, 1997), 140–45 passim.
2. Gay Hendricks and Kathlyn Hendricks, *Conscious Loving: The Journey to Co-Commitment*, (New York: Bantam, 1990), 100.
3. Ibid.
4. Richard Strozzi-Heckler, *The Anatomy of Change: A Way to Move Through Life's Transitions* (Berkeley, CA: North Atlantic Books, 1993), 79.

Index

labeling (meditation practice), 166–67

lactase, 127

lacto-ovo diet, 125

Las Vegas Convention Center, xiv

length (Center dimension), 311, 313–14

Leonard, George, 134

let-down headaches, 80–81

lifestyle: changes in, 136; as headache
  trigger, 55, 56–57, 71, 76–81

lighting, 71, 72–73, 77–78

light sensitivity, xvi, 5

lion's pose, 188

Little Circles (self-massage technique):
  basic instructions, 220, 221 *fig. 16-2*;
  benefits of, 220; in face self-massage techniques, 242, 243 *figs. 17-4,
  17-6*, 244, 248, 248 *fig. 17-11*; in head
  self-massage techniques, 237, 238,
  238 *fig. 17-1*, 239–40, 239 *fig. 17-2*, 240
  figs. 17-3a–17-3b; in neck self-massage techniques, 228, 229; in upper
  body self-massage techniques, 221,
  222

Little Frog Pads (Touch Prep technique): in face self-massage techniques, 242, 247–48; instructions
  for, 203–4, 204 *fig. 15-2*; as Mundo
  touch technique, 201; in neck
  self-massage techniques, 228; in
  upper body self-massage techniques, 220, 221

liver damage, 95

Lockheed Martin, xix

Look Far (loosening-up exercise), 191

Loosen the Hinges (Daily Breathing
  exercise), 146–47, 147 *fig. 11-1*

Low, Rodolfo, 103–5, 107

low-fat, high-carbohydrate diet, 127

luggage, 176, 180–81, 180 *fig. 13-5*

lunch, 120–22

Lying-Down Position (body position),
  291–92, 292 *fig. 19-6*

magnesium, 99, 113–14

maltose, 104

mandible, 247

MAO inhibitors, 67–68

massage: effleurage stroke in, 203–4;
  giver/receiver roles in, 207; use of
  term, 200. *See also* self-massage

Massage School of Santa Monica
  (CA), xvii

masseter, 247

Maxalt (triptan), 48, 93

maxilla, 247

May, Mitchell, 146

meals: frequency of, 108; healthy, planning for, 118; skipped, 65, 78; timing
  of, 109, 110

meats, cured, 67

medical procedures, 71, 88–89, 100

medication-overuse headaches, 15, 19,
  92–93

medications: caffeine in, 62, 109;
  mindful touch as alternative to, 199;
  tracking use of, 131

medication triggers: alternative therapies and, 98–100; dependence and,
  96–97; dosages and, 93–94; identify-
  ing/tracking, 92; MOH as result of,
  92–93; side effects and, 94–96; types
  of, 57, 91–92

Medina, Jose, 39

About the Author

*J*an Mundo didn't plan to become a headache healer, but in 1970 she learned she could relieve headaches, including her own, by putting her hands on the front and back of the head. From then on, no matter where she went, everyone seemed to know to go to Jan when they were suffering, and she would stop their pain.

Hundreds of headaches and twenty-one years later, she claimed her calling, became a certified massage therapist, trained in energy and intuitive work, learned about headaches and complementary medicine, and opened her practice in California. After receiving her first referrals from UCLA Medical Center in 1992, she was inspired not only to relieve her clients' pain but also to prevent it. With a keen interest in solving migraine mysteries, she translated her method into a touch protocol and designed a mind-body self-care program.

Motivated by personal health breakthroughs, she trained in mind-body therapies (qigong, breath work, mindfulness meditation) and — noticing how clients' emotional histories emerged with their pain — studied and earned certifications in Body-Centered and Conscious Relationship Therapy (Hendricks Institute) and Somatic Coaching (Strozzi Institute).

She has held programs and given lectures at medical centers, universities, corporations, and conferences, including Kaiser

Permanente Oakland, Hill Physicians Medical Group, UCSF Osher Center for Integrative Medicine, Stanford University, UC Berkeley, Lockheed Martin, Hewlett-Packard, Apple Computer, U.S. Association for Body Psychotherapy Annual Conference, International Headache Congress 2001, and New York Headache Center.

In *The Headache Healer's Handbook*, which she illustrated as well as wrote, Jan shares her nearly fifty years of headache healing wisdom. She is also published in the *Being Human at Work* anthology, *Massage* magazine, *Massage and Bodywork* magazine, the journal *Cephalalgia*, *Spiritual Midwifery*, and *The Farm Vegetarian Cookbook*.

Jan Mundo now lives and practices in New York City. She offers workshops, talks, and professional trainings nationally and internationally.

www.TheHeadacheCoach.com

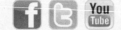